Praise for *Every.Single.Day.*

"This is one of those books that's inspiring not because the author wins the Olympics. But because she grabs the rudder of her own life, and steers a true, brave, and challenging course."

—Amby Burfoot, Boston Marathon winner, *Runner's World* writer at large

"What a pleasure to read Julie's transformative journey from a mile-a-day to a running expert in the space of a year. This book is not only a great documentation of true inner change, but it's full of wisdom, great running tips, awesome quotes and enough humor and encouragement to take anyone for as many miles as they want to go."

—Danny Dreyer, Author and founder of *ChiRunning*

"As a streaker for over 30 years, I understand what it takes to get the run in every day—no matter what! This is a great read for those wanting to get started streaking—or to get running period."

—Judy Mick, RRCA Certified
Running Coach, ASFA Certified
Running Fitness Instructor

"Insightful and often funny, this book details her struggles to find time for daily running, while juggling the demands of being a busy wife, mother, and writer."

—Mark Washburne, President,
Streak Runners International, United
States Running Streak Association

UNSTOPPABLE WISDOM FROM A YEAR OF RUNNING

EVERY. SINGLE. DAY.

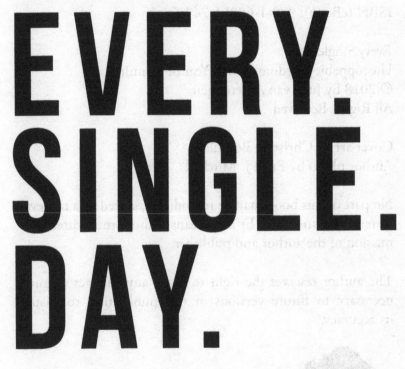

JULIE VAN AMERONGEN

PPRESS

A POST HILL PRESS BOOK

ISBN: 978-1-68261-748-9
ISBN (eBook): 978-1-68261-749-6

Every.Single.Day.
Unstoppable Wisdom from a Year of Running
© 2018 by Julie van Amerongen
All Rights Reserved

Cover art by Christian Bentulan
Author photo by Erica J. Mitchell

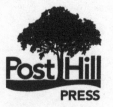

Post Hill Press, LLC
New York • Nashville
posthillpress.com

Published in the United States of America

NOTE TO READERS

A note to any of you thinking that you might like to try this at home: This is my story where I share information, inspiration, and, er…perspiration. I am not qualified in any way whatsoever to be a substitute for your doctor or healthcare provider nor do I or the publisher have any liability or responsibility to any person or entity with respect to any ill effects that may be incurred or alleged to have been incurred as a result of actions arising from the use of information found in this book. That is a long way of saying, use this information at your own risk. And I do hope you use it!

For Those Who Run,
And Those Who Aspire To

CONTENTS

CONTENTS

PROLOGUE

DAY 365. THURSDAY, MAY 5. PORTLAND, OR

Little by little a little becomes a lot.
—Tanzanian proverb

It feels like my birthday when I wake up today. I jump out of bed at dark o'clock and head out. OK, maybe I don't actually jump, but I'm moving with some extra umph, like I'm the holder of a special secret. Outside, the morning is mild and peaceful and on this run, like so many, I am reflective.

When I set out 365 days ago to attempt to run a mile a day every day for 30 days, truly I had no idea it would lead to this moment. I'd never heard of this kind of streaking and had no idea there was this amazing community of streak runners, all over the world, who have dedicated themselves to their health, fitness, growth, development, and their incredible support for one another.

I also had no idea I was capable of such a deep commitment to something that, while it serves me and the others around me so well, in many ways is all about me. I couldn't have known what it might be like to stick to this commitment no matter what was going on, where I might find myself, or how I might be feeling. I just didn't know what I didn't know. I had to create it myself.

I wondered for weeks whether this day's run, the one that makes one year of my running complete, would be dramatic and exiting or anticlimactic. It's not really either. I ran a handful of miles through my neighborhood, around the park and back like I'd done so many other times this year. No speed work, no hills, no company…just an easy run. Today's run isn't anything extraordinary which, I have learned, seems to be the way when you commit to something with such relentless consistency. This run, however, as part of that unwavering commitment to my running streak is a crucial brick in the wall of building something extraordinary—a solid, consistent, satisfying growth-builder of an experiment I am committed to Every.Single.Day.

For all the other streakers, my family who has supported me to get here, for all my unfolding and discoveries and for every literal step of the way here, I am so terrifically grateful.

Along the path in the park I find some chalk writing. It has an arrow pointing to the path and says, "You go, girl!" I believe I will. Streak on!

CHAPTER ONE

ABOUT STREAK RUNNING

Do it now.
Sometimes later becomes never.

What is a running streak? Nope, nothing to do with taking your clothes off here. Simply put, a running streak is running at least one mile within each calendar day—without fail.

According to Streak Runners International and the United States Streak Running Association, together the definitive authority on the subject, running may occur just about anywhere. Treadmills count (ellipticals don't). For the sake of my streak, at least one daily mile is defined as a continuous mile, without interruption for a stoplight, or a pesky shoelace.

The streak concept is somewhat controversial with a substantial group of naysayers who claim it is dangerous—that the implications of training consecutively without rest days can be deleterious to your health. Still, fierce advocates point to the implications of not training consecutively. If you take just one day off a week, that's 52 days of no training for a year. That's a lot of days.

Other than the minimum mile there are no other distance rules, and some runners cover considerably more distance than others. I have seen that as the distance increases so do the critics, exponentially. If it were so harmful I would think it would be hard to ignore so many people on the Streak Runners International list who have been doing this for years. Some for years and years, and years, and…years.

As for me, I have been enjoying the heck out of my streak, elevating the way I really listen to my body and providing myself with a good deal of variety in pace, distance, time and location. I think I was a good candidate for a streak because I was already running often—just not with true consistently.

Anyone considering a streak should probably give it some thoughtful consideration and consult with their healthcare professional as well.

CHAPTER TWO

THE JOURNEY OF 1,000 MILES

*The journey of a thousand miles
begins with a single step*
—Lao Tzu

In the early days of my career, I worked my way up from the front desk to the coveted Director of Marketing role at a hot start-up in lovely Marin County, California. When the company was sold, I got a severance package and some time to think. I wanted to put that marketing experience to good use in service of a product or brand I was really passionate about.

In Marin, there weren't a whole lot of eligible companies to choose from, but I wrote a letter and sent a résumé to a small handful and got a bite. The guy who reached out to me was a ball of energy—intense and direct, super smart and driven, yet warm and engaging too. I liked him immediately.

Just a few minutes into our conversation we cut to the chase and, from the same side of the table, Jeff and I began working together, not knowing that we would continue to do so…for the next 15 years!

When I say that, I mean that not a single day went by in all of those years when we weren't in touch multiple times a day—by phone, over email and/or in person, even on vacation or during holidays. Jeff was the single most prolific person I'd ever met. Period. I loved that energy and think we probably worked so well together because somehow, I could keep up with him.

As our work evolved over the years and our small team grew we added a right-hand man, a solid, reliable, consistently awesome guy. Kevin was so passionate about our mission, and no job was too big, too small, too above, or too beneath him. He did it all and he did it well, a lot of it in the pre-dawn hours of the day, the way he liked it. We were a good team.

One project Jeff and I collaborated on was a book called *Working for Good: Making a Difference While Making a Living.* During the process of writing the book, we interviewed a number of inspiring business leaders. Something I recognized in each of these highly successful people was a commonality regarding a personal practice or regular ritual of some sort that seemed to fuel them to show up optimally. Whether it was yoga or meditation or Tai Chi or surfing, every one of these leaders had an unwavering commitment to a practice they did regularly.

This nugget of information absolutely fascinated me, and I became a total practice geek, eventually launching The Practice Project, a series of interviews with conscious business leaders, artists, musicians, athletes, and others who all shared this non-negotiable commitment to their personal practices and for whom these practices were undeniably beneficial. As the project got off the ground, Jeff was the wind beneath my wings and Kevin was the webmaster and all around behind-the-scenes support.

Kevin and I had a regular weekly sit-down meeting. One week as we were meeting, he started patting his pockets like you do when you're looking for something. He'd somehow misplaced his phone and appeared flustered in a way I'd never seen before. After he located his phone he was still upset, unsettled, anxious…and I wondered if this is what a panic attack might look like.

A few minutes later, Kevin had the first seizure of his life. Within the span of an hour, he had gone from meeting with me to landing in the hospital where he learned that he had a tumor in his brain the size of a tangerine. A tangerine.

As if the tumor wasn't enough, Kevin soon learned he had glioblastoma. Google it and you will understand; there is no way around just how bleak it is. Without treatment, survival is typically just a few months after diagnosis. With treatment, the prognosis isn't much better.

Not one to take the news sitting down, Kevin jumped into action going full bore into research mode and any kind of alternative therapy he could get his hands on. We continued to work together as he could. In addition to the emotional strain, it was a challenging time at work. I'd come to really rely on Kevin and struggled both to keep the door wide open for his hopeful return to work and still get the work in front of me done.

Even though we might have known it was coming, when Kevin passed away months later it was still a shock and just so damned devastating. People in their 20s just aren't supposed to die. Thinking of the loss of his future, of what might have been…it was impossible not to be heartbroken. Still is.

Sad and shaken, two days after Kevin had passed I was walking out the door as the phone rings and I see from caller ID it is Jeff. I picked it up, eager to connect, but it was not Jeff on his own phone. It was a woman's voice. A voice that told me, "Julie, Jeff died."

Oh my God! Whaaaat? "Jeff died." My heart and my head struggled to reconcile what I'd just heard. Nothing about this made any sense.

Jeff was the most vibrant and robust guy around. He took exquisite care of his health. He surfed every day, ate really, really well, and just embodied the picture of good health. He was once the cover story for *Experience Life* magazine—wearing a smile and a suit while barefoot atop a surfboard. He was *that* guy. He traveled with his own blender to make his daily morning smoothie for crying out loud!

Jeff had had a heart attack in his sleep and died. He died just two days after Kevin.

It may sound cliché, but for me, the end of their lives was another beginning. In addition to coping with the heartbreak of losing both the amazing bright young light who was my right hand *and* my longtime constant companion, collaborator, colleague, partner, and dear friend, I was left holding the pieces of our business—and there was a lot to be done!

I did the only thing I really knew how to do: I just kept moving. It was something Jeff and I would often say to each other: "Just keep moving." It was a reminder both to move your body because that kind of movement begets other kinds of movement, and to keep your eyes on the prize despite the challenges. Besides, throwing myself even deeper into my work was a way of honoring both of them, right? Only it came at a cost.

I became increasingly obsessive about work. The volume of picking up midstream on so many things, looming deadlines and deliverables, and additionally dealing with the cold hard reality of the business of what happens when someone passes away, unexpectedly or not, was monumental.

A miserable fast track forward to a year after Jeff and Kevin had passed away I was at an all time low. I'd thrown myself so headlong into my work, and I was so tense and overcommitted, that I'd completely lost myself. The Practice Project had completely fallen off the map and I was all work, all the time, with little energy for **anything** else. I often wore the same thing for days in a row, a uniform of baggy jeans and a sweatshirt. I could just feel that when I did smile, the muscles in my face were heavy and unfamiliar. *I'd kind of forgotten how to do joy.*

Somewhere around this time, I saw a link for a television series: *The Tim Ferriss Experiment.* You might be familiar with Tim as the author of *The 4-Hour Work Week* and other books for hacking life, and I already a fan. His television series was all about mastery, taking deep dives into rich learning opportunities to do things he had always wanted to do but thought impossible.

In a week, Tim learned how to play drums and played live onstage in a huge theater with the classic rock band Foreigner. He mastered parkour, surfing, rally car racing, rapid language learning, and more. This is the kind of fun, creative, outside-the-box, cool, nerdy stuff I could totally grok on and the kind of stuff I'd already been learning and sharing through The Practice Project.

When I showed the series to my husband, Matt, he agreed that, yes, all of these things that Tim was accomplishing were amazing and inspiring, but…he wondered out loud whether Tim could manage this if he also had a partner or a family or even a dog! This eye opener raised a compelling question: What would an experiment like that look like for someone like me—a mom with a husband who travels constantly, busy kids, a full-time job, a 100-year-old house, a semi-neglected yard, a menagerie of rescue animals, and myriad other life responsibilities like almost every other middle-aged working mom out there, plus some lingering grief? Instead of "don't try this at home," what if I *did* try it at home?

I decided to experiment a little on my own terms to find out. I committed to a year of different 30-day practice challenges. A little step each day might just be something I could achieve and, if I could move it towards a bigger goal, that might be just the ticket to regaining the life I really wanted to be leading. It would be an exercise in controlling the things I could control. I figured that at the end of a year I would have tried a dozen different things, all of them long enough to potentially form a good habit and that perhaps I'd find a comfort zone again. I thought of the experiments as baby steps towards getting my mojo back—one challenge, one day, one *small* step at a time.

I started off with things I thought I could accomplish easily with that same kind of satisfaction you get from crossing things off a list. My first challenge started at home with clutter clearing. I picked up a copy of the outrageously popular book by Marie Kondo, *The Life-Changing Magic of Tidying Up*. I went through every drawer, cabinet, closet, room, and corner of my house and purged and cleared and cleaned and, as instructed, asked myself over and over if every single little thing I owned sparked joy. A lot of it did, and that felt good. A lot of it didn't, and massive amounts of boxes and bags, more than I could have imagined, exited my home. While almost always presentable, my homespace was now infused with freshness and really felt together. Progress.

I then took on 30 days of meditation. I'd always been a dabbler when it came to meditation, like one of those things you know is really good for you and you always feel better afterwards when you do it but you still have a hard time doing anyway. All this despite numerous retreats and years living across the street from one of the most well-known meditation centers in the country too! I'm somewhat embarrassed to admit this challenge was met with limited success, though the unexpected naps were a bonus!

I did accomplish 30 days of writing and 30 days of connection (reaching out and reconnecting with friends and family with whom I'd lost touch). I tried 30 days of logging my gratitude every day, 30 days of random acts of kindness, and 30 days of little things to jumpstart my mojo—anything from brushing my teeth with my non-dominant hand, walking a different route home from my office, letting my daughter pick my outfit, and so on.

In the mix of all of this and more, I took on the challenge of 30 days of running. Although I wasn't aware of the organization at the time, The United States Streak Running Association defines a running streak as "to run at least one mile within each calendar day. Running may occur on either the roads, a track, over hill and dale, or on a treadmill." I could do that, couldn't I?

I'd been a runner off and on for some time. I loved to run when I was in high school, but my ballet teacher, to whom I was devoted, frowned upon it. She said it would "ruin your long dancer lines." I ran a bit in college but got distracted by parties and following a certain band. I dabbled a bit in my early career days, but when my travel schedule looked like being away more than I was home, my running went out the window.

Ten years previously we were living in Track Town USA—Eugene, Oregon. There were bark chip running trails I could access right from my home and a whole community of people dedicated to getting out there. I began running in the early mornings inspired by so many other people who were doing this. It felt good and as a mom with two small kids, this was "me time"—my time and nobody else's.

With so much great running support around I committed to running a marathon. It had been on my bucket list forever. I trained with a group from the Eugene Running Company and loved every minute of it—honestly. I loved going for runs and thinking: "I have never run this far before in my life!" And, then doing it again the next weekend. And the next. I ran the inaugural Eugene marathon, and I still get teary eyed when I think about the way the crowd cheered us on. My name was on my runner's bib and people were shouting: "You've got this, Julie!" "Julie—way to go!" I was hooked. Only I wasn't.

I kept it up for a while, running a few days a week and running one more race after that, then I fell off the wagon… for several years. After a move to Portland, Oregon, I came back to running again. I found some other moms who were runners and we'd get out there before getting the kids to school.

I was back on the track. I was waylaid by injury. I ran. I loved it. I stopped running. I felt guilty. I ran. It was great.

I traveled and didn't run. The cycle went on. I was a runner again, but I still struggled with any kind of consistency.

During this time, my kids kept growing as they will do, and soon we started entering 5k races as a family. Admittedly, the promise of occasionally wearing some crazy costumes probably had us most excited, but the humanity of the crowd when hundreds or thousands or, in some cases, thousands and thousands of people get out there and run together is simply amazing. To this day, I don't think I've run a single race without getting verklempt (my family will also tell you that I cry at musicals and parades—yep).

More and more, running was a thing for us as a family, yet more and more I dabbled in and out of it. After Jeff and Kevin died I ran for sanity. I had a lot of days out there where it was the safest place to cry. Just keep moving and no one notices. But I also had a lot of days when I was just numbly planted in front of my computer. Day in and day out without any movement.

And so it was that in my attempt to gain my mojo back through this year of experimentation and 30-day challenges, I took on running every day for 30 days. Now, as I've explained, running wasn't new to me—but running every damned day sure was!

As I ran, day after day, something began to click, something that did not end at the completion of the 30-day challenge. It continues on to this day.

What follows next is a chronicle of what it was like, for me, to get my ass out the door Every.Single.Day. for a year. It's not sexy or, truthfully, even that captivating at times. It can't *all* be exciting if you do it every single day! What *is* exciting is the cumulative experience. This is simply just what happened when I put my foot out the door and one foot in front of the other…every day.

If you're someone who doesn't think they could do this, I think you're wrong. I did it and I possess no special talent or skill nor an abundance of free time or money or special equipment. You'll see. And, to all of the trail and ultra-runners out there for whom running my weekly distance and more in a single day on a regular basis is what you do…my hat is off to you all! You are amazing. Just wow. I am aspiring to be as badass as all that. But I am not there…yet.

This is the chronicle of what happened to me, just me. I wasn't trying to break any records or win any races, which is probably good because I didn't. I was just trying to transform my life, to figure out the way towards my joy again, to stay in shape, to see what I might be capable of and find out what would happen if I took something on and actually managed to stay with it on an unwaveringly consistent basis.

This is how I found myself moving out there on the road, the track, the trail and in some unexpected places and conditions…every day. Every.Single.Day.

CHAPTER THREE

EVERY.SINGLE.DAY.

As we run, we become.
—Amby Burfoot, Marathon Great

DAY 0.

There have been any number of periods in my life when the notion of running just one mile would have been laughable. "One mile?! But, I'm a *runner*. I've run a whole marathon—twenty.six.point.two.miles. You haven't even really begun to warm up at one mile!" Yet I find myself in a moment in time when my life feels so full, I'm struggling to fit in even a few miles—and to do it consistently. With running, like many other things, I've long held the notion that it's either all or nothing. So, when my life gets compressed...I don't run at all. *That is about to change.*

I am challenging myself to run (at least) one mile a day, every day for the next 30 days. That's all—one mile. Every.

Single.Day. It doesn't need to take a lot of time and you don't need to plan for it as much as you do with longer distances. It's the consistency I'm going for because that's what matters here.

DAY 1. THURSDAY, MAY 7. PORTLAND, OR

I step outside onto the front porch; it feels chilly and damp. I contemplate stepping back inside to just forget about it, and then I start to move. This is something I've done a million times before, right? My breath is a little ragged, then falls into that familiar pattern, if not a little heavier than usual. It's a rhythm I remember back to the days of long solo runs in high school. It's a beautiful spring morning, and I'm happy to be out. I'm back before I know it.

As my dear friend Jeff always used to say: "Movement begets movement." He was right. I am now moving through my day inspired and energized. Yes!

DAY 2. FRIDAY, MAY 8. PORTLAND, OR

Today I set out for 10 minutes but I run for 15 and it feels GOOD!

For me, running a few miles involves a time commitment minimally of about 45 minutes. You figure even at an easy pace (depending on your level, for most average runners that could look like six to 15 or more minutes per mile) you need to factor in some time to get dressed, run, cool down, and stretch or shower—so even if the running part takes you about 10 minutes for one mile, you need to consider the entire time it will *actually* take you to complete the whole cycle.

This is one reason I love running in the morning. I can get out of bed and put on my running clothes, run, stretch, shower, and get on with my day. If I run midday, I usually have to change whatever I'm wearing, think about timing my eating so my stomach is not so full as to give me a cramp but not so empty that I'm becoming too hungry, run, then shower—making it two showers in my day. That's a lot of extra time. When I don't run, I notice my performance and presence are diminished. That's reason enough to get out there, but as we all know, it's often not so simple as that.

TIP: Running in the morning is an incredibly efficient way to get it done and it really fuels me for the rest of the day. I feel like I've accomplished something first thing, it clears my head and gives me physical and cognitive energy for the day.

DAY 3. SATURDAY, MAY 9. PORTLAND, OR

I got my period yesterday, my head is foggy and my body is heavy. Before I realize what I have done this morning, I've eaten a full breakfast only to remember that my intention was to get my mile plus in first. Now my stomach is too full. Clearly, I've got a ways to go to re-establish my running habit, but committing to only a mile helps me remember I should be able to make the time at some point today.

In between my kids' soccer games I have a half-hour at home before I need to head out to the next one. What I really want to do is relax on the couch for a few minutes, respond to some e-mail, and have a tasty snack. What I do instead is put on my running shoes and head out.

It's a beautiful day, but my legs feel like they're carrying ankle weights (they're not) and I have a side cramp before I've gotten halfway down the block. Running in the afternoon means there are lots of people around and the interactions with neighbors and others make the time less contemplative and more interactive than I would typically experience in the early morning.

It wasn't really fun, but...I did it. And, I can swear that I would not have gotten my butt out the door without this challenge—and for that, I'm grateful.

DAY 4. SUNDAY, MAY 10. PORTLAND, OR

In strong contrast to yesterday, today I'm thinking that setting my sights on only one mile might not be rigorous enough. It's a beautiful morning. I go to the track and do my requisite loop (to the track with one lap and back to my house is about a mile) and my body is ready to do more. But my mind tells my body—"Hey, you don't have to. You can stop here and go home to the Sunday *New York Times* and a cup of tea on the couch before the kids get up." And so I do.

I later reflect that not pushing for more is not my usual way of undertaking something and wonder if this challenge needs some refining. Still, one mile down and four total for the week is four more than I probably would have done if I hadn't started this challenge.

TIPS THAT MIGHT HELP YOU GET OUT THE DOOR

- No matter what time of day you plan to run, **set out your clothes or pack your gym bag the night before.**
- For morning runners, **step out of bed and into your running clothes**—no fuzzy bathrobes or coffee in your pajamas here.
- **Resist the snooze button** or set your alarm for 15 minutes earlier than you usually do and indulge in the snooze just once.
- While easier said than done, at least for me, if you **get to bed earlier** it helps immeasurably too.
- **Resist the urge to sit down at your computer or check your phone before you go.** Until this year I'd lost many a morning run by checking my email while fully ready to run only to get sucked in by work that really could have waited until later.

Remember, you'll never regret going out for that run, but you may be cranky and unbearable to be around if you don't!

DAY 5. MONDAY, MAY 11. PORTLAND, OR

My husband, Matt, is still out of town, and the morning is compressed with a work project before I have to wake the kids and start the day in earnest. I work until 10 minutes before I need to kick into full gear with the kids and almost blow off the run. But...10 minutes is enough for one mile or so, isn't it? And, if I don't do it now, it's going to be really challenging to make it happen with my work and family schedule today. So, I throw on my running shoes. On the way out the door I notice our little dog looking guilty. Sure enough, she has apparently raided the bathroom garbage can and brought all the "treasures" back to her pillow. If I stop to take care of this business I will miss my chance to run.

I avert my eyes, go out for 13 minutes, jam through the door, clean up the mess, and make myself a mommy hero for the next 50 minutes—texting with the carpool, signing a permission slip, packing lunches, checking laundry, writing a couple of notes for teacher appreciation day, showering, dressing, and showing up for a meeting not one minute late. Phew—so grateful for that little mile!

DAY 6. TUESDAY, MAY 12. PORTLAND, OR

It's raining and it's cold, but I leave open a whopping 10–15 minutes for running after early morning work and before I need to move into full-on family morning mode. Matt is back in town, and he's game to join me. While we run we catch up and go through the day's family activities. We divide and conquer which one of us will attend the parent/player soccer meeting tonight and which one will be at the track meet, who will call the music teacher and who will follow up with the contractor we've been waiting to hear from, how we will manage picking up the present for the birthday party and who will check the online homework log and grading system for the kids and, and, and...multiple other things in 10 whole minutes.

My hands are cold and drops are running down my back, but we got in a short run *and* a family meeting and that feels good.

TIP: Running with a partner at an easy pace provides time for uninterrupted conversation. For some of us this might be the only time we get it!

DAY 7. WEDNESDAY, MAY 13. CHICAGO, IL

I'm out of bed at 4:15 a.m. to catch an early flight. I fly across the country. I have meetings. Matt flies in and meets me. We have room service in our hotel room with a nice bottle of prosecco. We are in a lovely sleep-deprived, bubbly wine-induced haze, and...we know we will feel better after a day of airplanes and canned air if we move, right? We head to the gym around 9:00 p.m. and knock out a few miles on the treadmill. It blows the cobwebs out from between my ears. I am *not* going to let travel derail my commitment this time!

Bad pun alert: Seven days without running makes one weak!

DAY 8. THURSDAY, MAY 14. CHICAGO, IL

Another super early morning—up at 5:30 a.m. Chicago time (3:30 a.m. Portland time if you are counting—and after an evening that included that wine), and running was just not going to happen this morning. After a nonstop day, we are super hungry. But...if we eat dinner first, it's less likely we'd get our mile or more in. So, we check in to our Airbnb, get a map of the neighborhood, and head out. We run on old concrete sidewalks, past restaurants, shops, crowded sidewalks filled with people smoking cigarettes, through a six-way intersection, and into a neighborhood.

My feet and body find the concrete completely unforgiving and it's raining, but I love seeing neighborhoods I would never see if we hadn't been on our feet. The run cleared my head and made me feel I'd really earned that most amazing Chicago-style pizza with an Oregon Pinot Noir (you can take the girl out of Oregon but…). Last time I was here in a similar setting, I had best intentions but only ran once during my four-night stay. This time **will** be different, guaranteed.

DAY 9. FRIDAY, MAY 15. CHICAGO, IL

Today is the closest I've come to cheating on the challenge. We walk on concrete sidewalks two and half miles to our seminar. After the full day there, we are walking back to our Airbnb and pass by a running shoe store. I've been wanting a new pair of running shoes for months. I love my Nike Airs, but the blessing and the curse of the more minimal style is how thin they feel when you walk or run on concrete, or on anything really, and mine have many miles on them. I pick up a new pair of the next model up with thicker (though still thin) soles and get a pair of gel-style inserts. I've never worn inserts before, and I worry about damaging my sensitive feet by being overly technical. They make my shoes heavier but if they will rid the balls of my feet of impact fatigue, I'm all for it.

We're hungry again and weigh the advantages of running before or after eating. Determined to get 'er done, we begin running *with* our backpacks and bags, dodging moving targets and the lines for seating at the outdoor restaurants. We're giddy at first, but it's humid out and our bags are heavy and

I feel like I'm late for a flight at an airport. We make it a half-mile before dropping that idea. We get to our place and that leftover pizza from last night is looking *really* good. In addition to the all-day seminar, we've walked five miles on concrete today, my feet are tired, and I'm starting to get hangry (for those not in the know, that's the crabby angry mode being hungry is responsible for).

Still, walking a handful of miles and running a half-mile doesn't count towards the challenge, so eyeing that pizza longingly, we throw on our running clothes and my new running shoes and head out. About 50 feet in, I tell myself how much I didn't want to do this a few minutes ago and how good the air feels and how glad I am that I'm doing it now. I can guarantee that this time I would have cheated had I not had Matt as my accountability partner urging us on for today's challenge. I'm proud of getting out and running at all, but especially in a new town.

TIP: Running outdoors while you travel is a great way to get to know a new place. Even just a couple of miles will show you something you wouldn't have seen otherwise.

DAY 10. SATURDAY, MAY 16. CHICAGO, IL

Yesterday was the closest I've come to cheating during this challenge, and today was the closest I've come to barfing. Another day of seminar, long walks on the concrete and a stop for some wine and tacos on our way back to our Airbnb. We drag our feet a bit after we get back but remind ourselves how quickly you can bang out a mile and how good it will feel to accomplish. At 10:00 p.m. we head out. This neighborhood is happening on a Saturday night, the weather is beautiful and people are out in full force. I have to laugh as I run by outdoor restaurants as people are drinking beer and smoking on the sidewalks. It's a fun way to experience a new place, but my feet are desperately missing the track or even blacktop instead of this concrete.

PROGRESS REPORT: 10 days. 10 miles. 10 entirely different experiences. Two cities. One new pair of running shoes.

DAY 11. SUNDAY, MAY 17. CHICAGO, IL

We were out the door by 6:30 a.m. this morning and in our seminar all day long. We debate knocking out a mile before heading to the airport but it's hot and humid and would seriously require a subsequent shower which we had no time for. We found our gate at the airport. Matt hung out with our luggage while I banged out a mile in Terminal 3, tracking it on MapMyRun on my phone. Then, I did the same for him.

When you run in an airport, dodging wheelie luggage and impacted Starbucks lines, you would think that people would assume you are late for a flight and get out of your way, but I can assure you now…no one does!

PS—O'Hare Airport—About those rotating plastic toilet seat covers…I feel like I'm sitting on a plastic bag that may or may not have been sat upon by someone else. How can those be anything but an environmental catastrophe anyway?! But I digress…

DAY 12. MONDAY, MAY 18. PORTLAND, OR

After being out of town for five days and arriving home late on a Sunday night, my Monday is jam-packed. I stay late at the office, and the rest of the evening is Boy Scouts and homework and laundry and the general catching up you need to do when you return home after having been away. By the time 10:00 p.m. rolls around it will be midnight in the time zone I'd adjusted to nicely over the last week, and I need to get my run in. I dread the idea of running at this time because the last thing I need before a well-deserved night of good rest is a pick-me-up, but…I head out. It's mild out, the air feels great, and I'm proud of myself when I'm done.

TIP: The hardest part is not the running. The hardest part is getting out the door.

DAY 13. TUESDAY, MAY 19. PORTLAND, OR

I run my mile first thing this morning. It takes little time, and it feels so good and like no big thing.

One of my favorite things to do after I run is to lay on the floor with my feet elevated in silence for a few minutes. The blood redistributes itself within my body, and it feels as if I am somehow integrating the run throughout my entire mind/body system. Like savasana[1] after a yoga class, it feels so good.

DAY 14. WEDNESDAY, MAY 20. PORTLAND, OR

At the two-week juncture I am struck by two things: I can guarantee that without the 30-day challenge I would not have gotten out every single day for a run, and…part of me wants to see if I can maintain this for a whole 365 days!

---

[1]   Corpse pose, the pose of total relaxation after yoga practice. Often one of the most challenging poses!

I haven't really run a distance longer than one mile in the last two weeks—something I probably would have done previously, just not consistently. Part of me wants to stop the challenge at 30 days to add some variety and distance. Then I realize nothing is saying I can't do both.

This is definitely an exercise for my body but it's almost more an exercise for my personal development, my determination and willpower.

It's also not lost on me that it is infinitely easier to bang out a mile when I am home. Travel continues to be an X factor that makes consistency exponentially more challenging. It's good to be home. My mile this morning is pleasant and will fuel me for the long day ahead.

DAY 15. THURSDAY, MAY 21. PORTLAND, OR

You can't flirt with the track. You must marry it.
—Bill Easton

My son, Shea, runs track. I have always enjoyed running but possess no particular talent. He, however, has been blessed with the gift of speed. As I run down to the track today to get my mile in I reflect on the race he runs—the 1500— three and three-quarter laps around the track, just shy of a mile. He runs it in a small handful of minutes. It takes two hands to count the number of minutes it takes many people to accomplish this feat and still others who need three, four, or more hands.

For me, it's not about my best time; it's just about getting out there and doing it. And, today, I do just that. Win.

DAY 16. FRIDAY, MAY 22. PORTLAND, OR

I am whupped this morning when I wake up and promise myself I'll run at some point during the day, then...I forget all about it. Matt is out of town, and it isn't until he forwards his MapMyRun tracker via e-mail that I remember I still have a run to get in.

I am surprised by how completely out of mind getting out for a run had been. Without that e-mail ping I might have completely forgotten and unintentionally blown the challenge!

Several hours later, though, I am still dragging and contemplate breaking the challenge anyway. Finally, I pull it together and head out the door. The transformation is almost instantaneous. They call exercise "nature's Prozac," and there is no doubt in my mind that is the truth. I had been feeling sluggish and just wanting to chill out or get to bed. Next thing I know I'm running up the middle of the street feeling almost euphoric. I wish I could bottle this transformative moment so I could use it to kick my own ass when I need it and to inspire others when they need it too.

DAY 17. SATURDAY, MAY 23. PORTLAND, OR

At this point in the game the novelty has worn off, and it feels like a bit of a chore. As soon as I am running it feels less so, but for the last couple of days it has felt more like an obligation than something I enjoy doing.

Then I remember that it doesn't matter if it's fast or slow, if it feels amazing or like a slog, the important thing is to do it. And to do it consistently. Seventeen days, baby!

*It seems to me, that for this task as well as much of life,
it's more than half the battle just to show up.*

DAY 18. SUNDAY, MAY 24. PORTLAND, OR

It's Sunday, and I get out first thing in the morning for a run in the neighborhood. I love seeing the newspapers piled up on the doorsteps, not yet collected by the sleeping occupants. Seeing other people out running or walking their dogs, you feel like part of a secret club of early risers.

Despite this, though, my run feels awkward. I'm not finding my stride even while adding in some extra distance. In fact, I recognize that not only am I not in better shape than when I started this challenge, I might even be in worse shape! My previous habit included running longer distances; the thing I struggled with was consistency.

*Right now, consistency is the real muscle I
am exercising. It's a little tight.*

Several years ago I was waylaid by a stabbing pain in my foot that was worsened by running. One day I saw a friend while he was out running. He asked why he no longer saw me out there on the road, and when I explained why he immediately recommended a podiatrist who specialized in running, Dr. Ray McClanahan. Dr. Ray had been a foot and ankle surgeon, performing hundreds of surgeries on his patients before realizing there had to be another way. He became convinced that the reason we were injuring ourselves running was because we'd strayed so far from the way our feet are naturally meant to be and our footwear had become overly technical and unnatural. To prove a point, Dr. Ray ran the Portland Marathon—in Crocs—and rocked it.

I went to see Dr. Ray and he diagnosed me with double neuromas. Neuromas are thickened tissue between the metatarsal bones of your feet that, when compressed, produce that icepick feeling. Interestingly, it also makes you feel like your socks are all lumpy under the balls of your feet when they definitely are not. He got me into some different footwear, and more importantly, got me *out* of some other footwear. I gave away literally thousands of dollars of shoes and reluctantly said goodbye to many pairs of lovely, lovely boots that were torturing my feet in order to start wearing footwear that was more natural—with a footbed actually as wide as my foot (try pulling the insole out of your shoes and watch the way your feet hang over the sides—yikes!) and toe boxes that allowed my toes to stretch out. I started wearing "Correct Toes," toe spacers that spread toes to a more natural and "correct" position and literally change your foot's shape.

Now I'm running, I've got some consistency, but shorter distance. To stretch myself I could work with my time—tracking my minutes and distance and charting my progress—and maybe I will.

Consistency requires discipline. And I know that with consistency and discipline I can accomplish anything I want.

DAY 19. MEMORIAL DAY, MONDAY, MAY 25. PORTLAND, OR

I learned about the United States Running Streak Association today. You have to run at least one mile every day for 365 days before you can actually join. Their active running list is continually updated. There is one man on the active running streak list who has not missed a day of running a mile a day for more than 45 years! Seriously. There are about 550 people on the list with a streak of at least one year and so many people who have done this for five, 10, 20, 30, 40 plus years! Wow. Wow. Wow. Amazing. Inspiring. Phew.

I guess all the streak runners who have come before me have passed the 19-day mark once!

I run in the late afternoon/early evening. It's a little bumpy finding a rhythm—it takes about a mile (I decide to run two). The weather is warm, and I am grateful for my healthy, fit body—and for all of those streak runners who log their miles and serve as inspiration to the rest of us.

DAY 20. TUESDAY, MAY 26. PORTLAND, OR

It's a beautiful night tonight and we take to some stairs for our mile.

My feet are killing me. Lately the pads under my feet feel like they've been in high heels all day—but that is definitely not the case. I know that as I have gotten older, the padding on the bottoms of my feet feel like it has gotten thinner. I haven't been comfortable going barefoot in years. But this soreness is new, and I suspect my new insoles have something to do with it. Time to gingerly experiment.

I say "gingerly" because neuromas, which have previously waylaid my running, are never far from my mind, and I do not take for granted being able to run on these small but mighty feet.

TIP: Nothing like sets of steep stairs to kick your butt (and legs and lungs). Phew.

DAY 21. WEDNESDAY, MAY 27. PORTLAND, OR

Tender feet call for a drive to the track to avoid the pavement and to share a beautiful, warm evening mile with my Matt and Shea. Shea laps us, and we admire his speed and stride. I just love getting out as a family even for a short bit with a healthy activity we all enjoy. This is one of those things that I hope our kids will remember about their upbringing when we are long gone. A perfect mile.

DAY 22. THURSDAY, MAY 28. PORTLAND, OR

Another drive to the track. Tonight I try experimenting with taking the inserts out of my new running shoes and find I'm a lot more comfortable. Is it really possible those inserts were harder on my soles and less shock absorbent than without them? The shoes are much lighter now, too, and my toes and feet feel relaxed and more comfortable than they have since I got the new shoes.

Another beautiful evening to be out after another full day of work and an afternoon/evening of activity. My time today could have been more effective if I'd gotten out the door first thing in the morning for the run. I remember how I woke to pee in the middle of the night last night because I drank more water than I usually do closer to bedtime after last night's run. I mull over these and other tradeoffs while I shower for the second time today, also not very time efficient.

I remind myself it's not always about being effective with my time but enjoying the time.

DAY 23. FRIDAY, MAY 29. PORTLAND, OR

Even though the evenings have been beautiful, I love getting the run in first thing in the morning. I don't have to think about it again for the rest of the day.

I run on the pavement without the inserts and my feet feel ok—a lesson to beware the overly technical running shoes. I am off for a very full day with my run under my belt and that always feels great!

PROGRESS REPORT: Days like today makes the concept of a longer running streak feel achievable. There's part of me that just doesn't want to break the momentum now. Only 329 (!) more days to make a year.

DAY 24. SATURDAY, MAY 30. PORTLAND, OR

Tonight marked the third running of the annual Starlight Run for our family of four. This is a long-standing costume run that uses the parade route of the Starlight Parade, one of the big attractions of the annual Portland Rose Festival. Since the run is just before the parade starts, the streets are lined with throngs of people cheering the runners on. The runners are so creative with their costumes, so festive, so friendly, and there are so many—all running the three-plus mile route.

For me, it is one of those experiences that makes you feel hope and love for humanity. It's become a tradition we look forward to all year long.

The evening is beautiful, warm with a colorful sunset. It's not a timed run and even with the hills, each one of us knocks it out with ease buoyed on by the energy of the other runners and the crowd. Such a fun, happy, healthy tradition that I'm so grateful to share with my family. The family that runs together stays together!

DAY 25. SUNDAY, MAY 31. PORTLAND, OR

Ordinarily, I might take a day off of running following a race to allow my body time to recoup, but a 5k isn't a long race. Still, in honor of taking it a bit easy, Matt and I run with the dogs. They love to run, but we don't always love to run with them as their frequent stops to take care of nature's call and to bark at squirrels or sniff other dog butts cramps our style. But for today, we run with them and frolic together all over the dog park. My feet are happy to run on the grass and we are all happy to play together. Running *and* running the dogs—check.

DAY 26. MONDAY, JUNE 1. PORTLAND, OR

What a day! Early-morning obligations and a very full work-day. I work late and eat dinner in the car to get to a meeting on time. By the time I land at home for the night and take care of a few things, I am pretty wiped out.

Shea asks me what happens to a running streak when someone gets sick, but I am not ready to find out. For now, it's after 10:00 p.m., drizzling and chilly, but Matt and I bang out our mile plus a little more. Even though many experts would tell you not to exert yourself before bedtime if you want to sleep, I don't think that mile is going to have any impact on my dreamtime tonight.

PROGRESS REPORT: Five more days to complete the 30-day challenge, and I am already clear that I'm not stopping there. I'm getting so much out of it there's no giving up now.

DAY 27. TUESDAY, JUNE 2. DENVER, CO

Another travel day, another late night run in a hotel gym. A run is just what the doctor ordered after sitting in the middle seat of the plane for hours. Arriving at the gym, Matt and I are surprised to have this massive place all to ourselves, and even better—no crappy, pumping music blaring through the speakers. We are five minutes into our treadmill run when security arrives to tell us the gym closed over an hour ago! We ask if we can stay for a few more minutes, and they graciously oblige. Wanting to be considerate of their time I attempt to set a personal record on the gym equipment so that we can hit the mile mark and leave quickly.

I remember a time when I used to travel and not pack any workout clothes. Those days are long gone. Tonight's run was silly and fun, adding a dimension of adventure to our travel.

TIP: Pack your workout clothes when you travel, no matter what. Queue up a workout video, stick some exercise resistance bands in your bag…anything to lower the opportunities to make an excuse not to exercise.

DAY 28. WEDNESDAY, JUNE 3. DENVER, CO

An early start to a long day that ended with a wonderful dinner with friends and colleagues over several shared bottles of wine. We get back to our hotel—we haven't stepped foot here in 15 hours. Not long ago that would have been it for me—I'd have been in for the night. But it's closing in on midnight with only a fleeting window of time to get the run done on this day. The gym, as we now know, is closed for the night. We head out the hotel driveway, down the road, and into a park. Somehow, even though we are stuffed and full of wine, the run is easy to bang out, and we appreciate the park space and new adventure. A win.

PROGRESS REPORT: 28 days. Three states. Two hotel gyms. One run inside an airport.

DAY 29. THURSDAY, JUNE 4. PORTLAND, OR

Matt and I are wiped from a day of travel, then work, kid activities and getting caught up at home. It's a mild night and after dinner I'd like to take a walk and not run, but we head out to run around 9:30 p.m. anyway. I immediately have upper and lower side stitches on both sides of my ribcage on account of having eaten so recently. Matt and I hobble along through the park. He asks: "How much longer until this challenge is over?"

I answer truthfully that we're almost on Day 30 and that I'd like to keep the challenge going longer, but I feel less convinced than I've been lately.

Then I notice…did I just catch myself complaining?! I met a man this afternoon who suffered a stroke three years ago. It took an entire year for him to learn to walk again. He told me that when he started walking without his walker that he must have fallen down 200 times. I said he must have gotten up 201 times. So what if a run today isn't my favorite? I can run. End of story.

DAY 30. FRIDAY, JUNE 5. PORTLAND, OR

The weather is beautiful, and there are more people in the park in the early morning than usual. In the winter the outdoor tennis courts are barren, but this morning, they are hopping. We run into several friends and have some lovely conversation and connection. A mile plus social time to start the day.

I'm not sure what I thought would happen in 30 days, but I'm finding this entire experience a compelling and eye-opening exercise in stretching my dedication and consistency muscle, as well as experiencing something old in an entirely different new way. I am having fun and think I am growing and re-finding some of my old self. Can't wait to see what the next 30 days brings!!

DAY 31. SATURDAY, JUNE 6. PORTLAND, OR

A long and busy day forces the run to happen in the evening. It's warm, and we run with the dogs to and around the park. I love running in the grass, perhaps not as much as they do, but a lot. The tufts of grass cushion my feet as they strike, and the differing terrain really makes you have to stay on your toes—metaphorically and otherwise.

DAY 32. SUNDAY, JUNE 7. PORTLAND, OR

Another long, hot, busy day. Another evening run with the dogs in the dog park. They're happy. We're happy. We run into friends with their dog on the way home. They love the mile-a-day challenge idea and ponder what it might be like for them. We highly recommend they give it a try.

DAY 33. MONDAY, JUNE 8. PORTLAND, OR

11:00 p.m. rolls around, and I am getting home after an endless day of work and meetings. So grateful I knocked out a quick and easy run to start the day. Today it felt as if there were nothing to it, and I will take that for the win!

DAY 34. TUESDAY, JUNE 9. PORTLAND, OR

This is the last week of school for the year, so in addition to typically full work schedules, every night includes year-end gatherings and exhibitions, graduations, parties, etc.

It's supposed to be another hot one and a very full day ahead so I make time to run first thing in the morning. I am fueled for the day!

DAY 35. WEDNESDAY, JUNE 10. PORTLAND, OR

I could get used to this quick and easy morning run routine!

Another compressed day ahead, another beautiful morning, another day charged up by my morning run!

DAY 36. THURSDAY, JUNE 11. PORTLAND, OR

I think I know now that the reason they tell you to wait to go swimming for half an hour after you eat is not because you'll drown but because you might throw up in the water!

My belly full of pizza, we go for a night run. Matt suggests we run two miles—one right before midnight, the other after so we get a mile in on both days. It's clever, but I think it would be cheating. We go for a mile plus and try to ignore what is happening with the pizza as we enjoy the night air.

DAY 37. FRIDAY, JUNE 12. PORTLAND, OR

Even while I enjoy the evening runs, morning time is where it's at. I run and then I don't think about having to do it again all day long.

Running gets me out and going this morning—like a natural cup of coffee. And then I am done!

DAY 38. SATURDAY, JUNE 13. PORTLAND, OR

I'm heading across the country by plane and know my day will be filled with an inordinate amount of minutes spent sitting on my butt. This makes getting out for some serious exercise today an imperative so I am especially grateful that I got in my run this morning before taking off. My running gear is packed and ready to go!

DAY 39. SUNDAY, JUNE 14. ARLINGTON, VA

I ran into a friend the other day who is a serious runner and told him about our mile-a-day challenge. We discussed how running while you travel can be a great way to get to know a place. He told me about the last time he was in the city he'd grown up in yet a 12-mile run showed him all kinds of secret places he had never seen before.

Matt and I are sharing a run this morning in Arlington, Virginia, and I can attest that even a couple of miles is helping us to get to know a whole new side of the place that we're visiting. Winning.

A NOTE ABOUT SOCKS

I really love the extra padding of **Thorlo cushioned socks**, and I find them super comfy. A lot of distance runners stick to pure wool to keep blisters at bay, but as long as I'm not running too long or too hot, I'm a big fan of these multi fiber socks.

I've recently added a rainbow of **DryFit socks** to my collection and am loving them too. They have a non-cotton padded sock that is becoming a favorite.

Smartwool. Wool has a reputation for warmth, which is not always what you want in your running socks, but these super thin wool/nylon socks are recommended for moisture management. I like the fit, and they're durable and not warm like you might think.

I've also experimented with compression by adding pairs of **Zensa** and **CEP calf compression sleeves**. They make my legs feel springy, but I'm not 100% sold on the benefits and if you had been a fly on the wall watching me getting them on and off you would know that can be a serious workout in and of itself too!

DAY 40. MONDAY, JUNE 15. ARLINGTON, VA

Another day and another side of this lovely neighborhood. Interesting to note—there are no sidewalks here! The story goes that when these neighborhoods were originally built the lack of sidewalks presented a favorable upscale image for the neighborhood. Ironically, walking was déclassé and driving was the bomb! The streets are wide, and it's not hard to move to the side to let cars pass but I do find I miss the false sense of security a nice sidewalk will present when necessary.

DAY 41. TUESDAY, JUNE 16. WASHINGTON, DC

Running in the hotel gym is not a great way to see the city, but it is a handy place to bang it out before you go and do so. Done and done.

DAY 42. WEDNESDAY, JUNE 17. BALTIMORE, MD

In Baltimore, some of the city parks are so big that all we have to do is run to the other side of a freshly mown field and back again to hit our first mile. A nice path along a little river (or is it a big creek?) gives us some extra miles in the shade on a hot and humid morning. Once again, running while traveling is proving to be a great way to get to know part of a place you might not see otherwise and today is no exception.

DAY 43. THURSDAY, JUNE 18. CROTON-ON-HUDSON, NY

During our travels, we stop at the Croton Dam in Croton-on-Hudson, New York, the town I grew up in. It was once known as the tallest dam in the world, built in the late 1800s. A park and beautiful trails surround this stunning and remarkable place. It is actually the largest hand-hewn structure in the U.S., and third only in the world after the Great Pyramid of Giza and the Great Wall of China.

After hours in the car, a run is a great way to recharge the batteries. We run from the lower park to the top of the bridge for the views. I am nostalgic for my childhood as I remember many happy days spent frolicking in the park and some angsty teenage days, too, spent pacing around the park with David Bowie blaring through my Sony Walkman. Running was a fantastic way to revisit an old place, introduce it to my family, and get in some great views to boot.

DAY 44. FRIDAY, JUNE 19. EAST FISHKILL, NY

Visiting the new weekend home of some relatives in New York, our run is along a dirt road that reminds me of the road I grew up on as a child, and on which I first started running when I was in high school. The flora and landscape is the same. When I stop to snap my usual quick photo, I attract a swarm of mosquitos.

TIP: Running fast is a good way to keep pesky mosquitos away!

DAY 45. SATURDAY, JUNE 20. EAST FISHKILL, NY

We are surrounded by a swarm of horseflies today during our run. They are *everywhere*! We run fast, slapping at our backs and shooing the air. Then we see a fox darting away with a squirrel in its mouth—a sight that makes dealing with those horseflies more than worthwhile. Yes!

DAY 46. SUNDAY, JUNE 21. NEW YORK, NY

It warms my heart to see the hotel gym so full of people early in the morning on a Sunday. I know how my workout fuels me for the day and imagine people everywhere fueling up for a dynamic day while other people are still sleeping. Plus,

the views from this gym, on the top floor of our hotel, are
pretty sweet.

DAY 47. MONDAY, JUNE 22. NEW YORK, NY

We walked all over Manhattan yesterday doing so many
things and I felt just great, energetic and healthy all day long.
I attribute a good deal of that to the energy I got from our
morning run and am glad to get another one in here this
morning to prepare me for another full-on day of touristing
in my old home city.

DAY 48. TUESDAY, JUNE 23. NEW YORK, NY

I watch the window washers high up on platforms while I
run on a high-tech treadmill that seems more robust than
the scaffolding out there. I hope those folks are well com-
pensated and well insured! The setting is fun and so different
than what I experience during a typical run at home.

PROGRESS REPORT: I've completed a 10-day vacation and ran
every day of it. I am amazed at how something that used
to feel like such a challenge—exercising while vacationing—
was no big deal and am grateful for how healthy and vibrant
I felt along the whole way.

DAY 49. WEDNESDAY, JUNE 24. PORTLAND, OR

Running down the street this morning I am struck by how
relatively easy it is to bang out a few miles on a machine at
the gym versus hitting the real road. It feels much more chal-

lenging to propel myself forward as I get started this morning, first time back outside in a few days.

As I run, Portland feels like a Podunk town compared to Manhattan. School let out just before we left for our trip. Now the park, in the early morning, is filled with parents shuttling their kids to swim team at the outdoor pool, tennis lessons, boot camp on the soccer field, and people walking their dogs. I want to stay at the track longer but I have a big day ahead. The run keeps my head fresh during our first day back—a long day at the office and a late-night entertaining at home.

DAY 50. THURSDAY, JUNE 25. PORTLAND, OR

I'm reminded this morning how quickly you can run a mile when that's all you have the time to do. I have a conference call in half an hour. I head out for a flat, straight mile, jump in the shower, eat a quick breakfast, and make my call on time. Perhaps just one mile isn't a tremendous workout, but it's done and leaves the day open for more; if not, this much at least is under my belt.

DAY 51. FRIDAY, JUNE 26. PORTLAND, OR

If you are planning to run, figuring out what to eat and when can be a challenge. There seems to be a magical formula for what fuels each runner best—how much and what they eat, how long before they run and how they hydrate. As you get into longer and longer distances this becomes a big deal—along with when you have to go to the bathroom!

My magic formula for my morning run is to have nothing but a glass of water upon waking before heading out shortly thereafter. If I wait much longer I begin to get hungry and then just don't have the stamina to maintain the pace and distance I desire. This morning, I wait a little too long to get out the door and I feel it. Still, I'm happy to get out and tomorrow I'll do it sooner upon waking.

Matt is out of town today. His flight yesterday was cancelled, and he took a late redeye, got to his destination just in time, performed all day and was texting me to say goodnight when he realized he hadn't gotten his mile in. He got out of bed, got in his mile, and got back in bed. Phew.

DAY 52. SATURDAY, JUNE 27. PORTLAND, OR

Fy vay em? What is this thing you call fy vay em?
—People who don't understand early risers

It's Saturday and I awake at 4:45am because I am so warm. It's supposed to hit 100 degrees here today, and it still hasn't cooled off from yesterday. I am up and about and out for my run by 5:00 a.m. Already there are others at the track, and a couple of the tennis courts are in action. I love rising early and getting the run in to have a spacious morning stretching out in front of me before it gets hot.

DAY 53. SUNDAY, JUNE 28. PORTLAND, OR

I postpone my morning run so Matt and I can run together since he is flying home later. Due to the heat we don't get out until late evening. The air is cool and the run feels great. It's long enough after dinner so my stomach isn't full; I feel I can go and go.

DAY 54. MONDAY, JUNE 29. PORTLAND, OR

Up and at it early today. It's going to be another hot one. We ran so late last night and so early this morning; it's like having a sleep sandwich. No matter; it's a wrap!

DAY 55. TUESDAY, JUNE 30. PORTLAND, OR

Matt has an early flight today and we get our run in before he takes off. Any day that starts with a run is better than any day that doesn't—especially when that day means sitting on a plane all day.

As I run I reflect that 55 days feels like a lot of days but 310 more to make a whole year still feels like a lifetime away!

DAY 56. WEDNESDAY, JULY 1. PORTLAND, OR

This morning my time is compressed. I run just a hair over a mile and it takes not much more than 10 minutes. I reflect on the many ways in which I spend 10 minutes in my day— on a call, in a meeting, making lunch for the kids, and the many ways I might waste 10 minutes—on the line in the grocery store, scrolling social media, and so on.

Even a 10-minute run can have a significant impact on your day.

How many other ways could I spend 10 minutes in my day that would have such a positive impact on me or my family or my work environment or community? Ten minutes is long enough to make a difference.

DAY 57. THURSDAY, JULY 2. PORTLAND, OR

We're in the middle of a heat wave. It doesn't usually get this hot this consistently here. Many people in Portland live in lovely old houses with old heating systems and no air-conditioning—myself included. It was so hot last night that I slept in the basement where it's cool and dark, and…missed hearing my alarm in the morning. I woke with a start. It's been so many years since I've overslept that I can't remember the last time. In short, no time for a run this morning.

It's still 98 degrees when I get home from work at 6:00 p.m. I am not someone who thrives when it's this hot out, and I am not ready to run outside in this heat!

I'm tired and cranky from the heat, working long hours, and solo parenting this week, and I have my period and a budding headache. I'm seriously about to Google mothers + working full time + husbands who travel + mental health when I remember I still haven't run. Sh*t. I head out at 11:00 p.m. The kids are still awake as the heat keeps us all up late. It's still 84 degrees out at 11:30 p.m., and I haven't eaten dinner yet.

A lot can happen in a run. I see some new street art that warms my heart and run alongside a woman I have seen running in the neighborhood for years, amazingly not wearing anything reflective on a dark night either, like me. The breeze feels good. It's cooler outside than in. I'm still a little cranky, but at least I didn't break my streak!

DAY 58. FRIDAY, JULY 3. PORTLAND, OR

The heat keeps me up late and wakes me early. I'm up by 4:30 a.m. and don't want a repeat of yesterday's experience so

I am out the door by 5:00 a.m. It's even warm now, but it's pleasant and now…I am done!

DAY 59. INDEPENDENCE DAY, SATURDAY, JULY 4. PORTLAND, OR

Heading out for a run before heading out for a hike feels counterintuitive, but we're going for a waterfall hike with the masses to beat the heat and I know I won't be running there, so off we go. Run done and I feel great on the hike too.

DAY 60. SUNDAY, JULY 5. PORTLAND, OR

The heat is still happening. Early runs are the way to go because there's not another time in the daylight hours to make it happen comfortably. This week I am not breaking any speed or distance records but I am maintaining a consistency record.

How many other ways could my life change if I were this consistent with other habits?

DAY 61. MONDAY, JULY 6. PORTLAND, OR

During my run on this mercifully cool morning, I reflect how I have enthusiastically started a lot of things in my life: art and home projects, hobbies, small businesses and websites, and so on, only to have my interest wane when the novelty wears off and it requires real diligence to remain focused.

Like many things worth pursuing, this challenge is almost less about the activity itself and more about relentless forward progress

This is about proving to myself that I can stick with something beyond the fun and the novelty, and that I can keep myself in good shape, enjoy myself even when I resist, share the time with Matt and others, set a good example for my kids and set the bar for other challenges in my life just a little bit higher.

DAY 62. TUESDAY, JULY 7. PORTLAND, OR

Matt is running a little slow today and I can tell he is going gingerly—not in pain, but watching it.

We all seem to have things we need to watch for; for me, it's my feet, for Matt, his knees, for others it's their backs, etc. One thing I appreciate about this challenge is that if you choose to do just the mile or so, it's a reasonable request. The consistency helps support a level of maintenance and satisfaction that doesn't push us into the danger zone of overtraining by doing too much, too hard without building up to it. I am uber-cautious in this department not wanting to risk being waylaid by my precious and sensitive feet.

PROGRESS REPORT: I love a good challenge, but even with 62 days in, 303 more days to make a year feels precarious. One day at a time as they say.

A thoughtful approach to running and a book by the same name called *Chi-Running* advocates for a running technique transformation that includes landing with a midfoot strike (I changed from a heel strike several years ago and have never looked back) and using proper alignment, posture, and a forward lean to reduce injuries and improve performance. My pal Jeff helped to bring this book to life. I'm a big fan and recommend checking it out.

DAY 63. WEDNESDAY, JULY 8. PORTLAND, OR

I'm on a roll where banging out a couple of miles or more *every* day feels like no big whoop. By the end of the day I can hardly remember that I started it with a run—though I suspect it would be quite conspicuous in its absence and effect on my days. I feel healthy, strong, and consistent. Now if only running would sculpt my arms the way it does my legs!

DAY 64. THURSDAY, JULY 9. PORTLAND, OR

Today's theme: What more am I capable of?

Yesterday I imagined that it was getting easier to run consistently, perhaps because our summer schedule is a wee bit more spacious than during the school year. Yet this morning there are orthodontist appointments for the kids, an extra-early morning conference call, cat puke on my computer keyboard, and a flight to catch along with all the other usual activity of any busy family with full-time work and travel to boot. And…the run still feels like no big deal. Perhaps it is not.

Perhaps my capacity has expanded for making this happen not just periodically but with daily consistency—not to the detriment of anything else but with the magnitude of accepting other daily challenges.

DAY 65. FRIDAY, JULY 10. PORTLAND, OR

Any long distance runner will have stories for you about going to the bathroom in unexpected places. You get out there on a long haul with everything jumbling around, the urge strikes and you have no choice but to heed it. During the 1998 London marathon, they called winner Catherine McKiernan's condition "stomach cramps." At the 2005 London marathon winner Paula Radcliffe stopped by the side of the road in full view of the crowds and TV cameras desperate to deal with her diarrhea. I'll leave it to your imagination as to why this is the theme of today's run!

DAY 66. SATURDAY, JULY 11. PORTLAND, OR

The other day I was thinking about the race up the stairs at the Empire State Building and how it might be fun to do something like that—something different, challenging, but that's over quickly. Then today I threw some stairs into my morning run, and I changed my tune. Holy moly—running stairs, real staircases, is nothing like being on one of those stairsteppers at the gym! Running stairs is grueling. I know I shouldn't be so surprised, but talking and doing are entirely different things. I'm ready to add more variety to my runs, increasing my strength and stamina, but I am clearly not ready to take on the Empire State Building any day soon. Phew.

DAY 67. SUNDAY, JULY 12. PORTLAND, OR

This morning I'm running with my boy, which makes me so happy. Getting this teenager out of bed early on a Sunday morning is actually a much bigger feat than the run itself. I love running at tempo pace[2] and our ensuing conversation, more spacious than conversations at home or with others around. We pass some neighbors and friends in the park and I feel proud to be running together. For the final block of the run, we sprint. I surge ahead to start us off and am quickly overtaken, clearly no big deal for this guy. I feel like a zebra being taken down by a lion. I remember playing tag when he was younger and the days when I could go head to head with him in a race—lifetimes ago, but just as much fun now as then.

DAY 68. MONDAY, JULY 13. PORTLAND, OR

I was on my feet and walked many miles yesterday and feel heavy in the legs and foggy in the head this morning and… the morning run just knocks the cobwebs right out. It isn't perfect, or faster, or longer, or vastly different than any other run. Just appreciating that what feels like little effort has such a nice return in the moment, for the remainder of the day and overall in general. Winning.

---

2   Tempo pace is runner speak for running comfortably hard, a pace you could maintain for a while.

DAY 69. TUESDAY, JULY 14. PORTLAND, OR

Good weather and no travel make the perfect storm to get out consistently. Day 69 and in a pleasant holding pattern.

DAY 70. WEDNESDAY, JULY 15. PORTLAND, OR

More beautiful weather and excellent morning running conditions. I am on a roll!

But before I pat myself on the back too hard…I note that I somehow seem to have forgotten that this started out as a 30-day challenge and have now pointed myself towards the 365 day mark. In 297 more days it will be mid-May of next year. That's still a lot of small steps towards a year's worth of consistency. If you make it injury, illness or obstacle-free… then what happens? After a year do you just go back to your old ways? Only time will tell! Meanwhile, it feels a worthwhile and thankfully fun exercise.

DAY 71. THURSDAY, JULY 16. PORTLAND, OR

I made an error this morning that I used to make all of the time. I'm up, I'm out of bed, I'm dressed for my run, and… then I start diving into my inbox to answer a few e-mails before preparing for my first meeting of the day. One e-mail leads to another and the next thing I know I am right up against my time limit. Ready to run but out of time. This is the first time this has happened in almost 70 days and the best part is that unlike previous times when this would have meant that my chances of running during that same day were over, I now have a relentless daily commitment to fit it in, no matter what. I go out for a lunchtime run. It's usually not my favorite time, but today it's a good comma in a jam-packed day.

DAY 72. FRIDAY, JULY 17. PORTLAND, OR

I love going somewhere where somebody is mouthing off
about how much money he makes or how important he is,
and I don't say anything, but inside I'm thinking,
"The only thing that's in shape on him is his mouth!"
—Doug Mock

Not wanting a repeat of yesterday's timing, I'm up and at 'em early banging out a loop that includes a set of stairs. This is not the Empire State Building, but I'll consider it a win.

DAY 73. SATURDAY, JULY 18. PORTLAND, OR

I'm taking my morning run with Shea this morning, which I just love. Anytime I can spend one-on-one doing something we both enjoy together is a bonus in my book. Add to that the good news waiting in my inbox when we return from the run—an invite from his track coach to attend summer running camp. As an incoming high school freshman this is an honor and an auspicious way to begin his high school career. How fortunate he is, and what a great, challenging, growth experience it will be!

DAY 74. SUNDAY, JULY 19. PORTLAND, OR

It seems timing is everything in setting the right conditions for a run. Today, we did what we could but our timing is not ideal, getting out sandwiched between games at my daughter

Calliope's soccer tournament on a 100-degree day. Matt manages to pant this: "hot…hungry…." But afterwards, no regrets.

DAY 75. MONDAY, JULY 20. PORTLAND, OR

Better timing today. Up and out first thing in the morning on this beautiful day. An easy run and a laugh shared with neighborhood parents whose kids are away at summer camp with ours. This sure makes getting out for a run and accomplishing myriad other things easier—and we can talk about how we miss them while we do!

It may be time to take on one more additional daily challenge. My lower body is strong and fit—the upper, a little wimpy, like a T-Rex.

What does it take to commit to another daily addition to your routine? It is, actually, a big decision. The occasional time is no big deal, but the daily consistency is a whole other thing!

DAY 76. TUESDAY, JULY 21. PORTLAND, OR

Matt's knee is tweaked this morning. He has to take it really easy on our run. I suspect that whatever is bothering him is not related to our daily mileage but to other exercises provided by a trainer that he does with intensity, but sporadically.

Injury scares the h-e-double toothpicks out of me. Being waylaid from running due to foot pain quite literally changed my life. I was a different person when I had no outlet for my physical energy. My energy, stamina, cognitive function, and general approach to life were all affected. Here's hoping for a quick recovery and more caution moving forward!

DAY 77. WEDNESDAY, JULY 22. PORTLAND, OR

On the way out the door this morning, we run into a neighbor who immediately asks, "You're going running? What are you training for?" The assumption is clear—you're going out, there must be an end in mind, and likely a competitive one at that. It sparks a good conversation about the varied ways we can approach running—or really anything. Sometimes we're in training for a big goal. Sometimes we're laying the groundwork for that training. Sometimes we're just engaged with the practice for no other purpose than that.

I am mindful that training for a goal without the habit of consistency is a good recipe for injury. Today I am in training for the long-term habit of consistency in running and in life. Period.

DAY 78. THURSDAY, JULY 23. PORTLAND, OR

Matt's knee is still bothering him so he heads to the gym to get his mileage in on a machine while I opt for the fresh air. During the run I reflect about the reason why people aren't consistent with their good habits, whatever they might be— running, eating right, and so on.

On the outside, consistency isn't sexy. It's predictable and kind of boring. I don't think many people aspire to that. Yet what is sexy is that consistency wins. It gets the best results. It just works. Willingness and consistency, like slow and steady, wins the race.

DAY 79. FRIDAY, JULY 24. PORTLAND, OR

It's a beautiful morning for a quick, easy run before my first meeting of the day. Not sexy but pretty fun actually as I tried out a new route. I'm trying to remember the last time

I committed to anything beyond my daily essential habits that I have done consistently for this many days in a row without stopping and, honestly, I'm having trouble coming up with much.

Years ago I gave up alcohol for a month, which turned to a year and then two-plus years. I hadn't been a big drinker but it was a couple of years of going to parties and drinking sparkling water. After a while I forgot I was "doing" something. It was just the way it was. This running pattern, now that I am not traveling and the kids are off for the summer especially, feels that way too.

But honestly, the fact that I can't come up with anything else I have relentlessly committed to like this makes me a little sad, mad, and determined to do more.

Matt is pondering the same thing. He decides not to run today because the tweak in his knee is present and asking him to pay attention. He started this challenge with me after I was a few days in and he's been my companion whether in person or one of us is on the road, sending each other our MapMyRun tally for the day. I'm sad for the break for him but respect how important it is to listen to your body. And, I'm grateful that I feel good and plan to continue on as long as I can.

DAY 80. SATURDAY, JULY 25. PORTLAND, OR

This has been the hottest summer I can ever remember around here, and everything is dusty and dry, so the mist in the air this morning feels awesome. I run to the park and around the track. There are all kinds of early morning park activities—community soccer games, tennis, swimming—

and everyone seems to be loving the smell and the feel of the moisture in the air.

About halfway into my second mile I get some unfamiliar and wicked stomach cramps. Could it have something to do with the crazy late-night combo of wines and cheeses I had at the Wine with Dogs gathering (yep—who knew?!) we unexpectedly stumbled upon? Why yes, it probably does.

DAY 81. SUNDAY, JULY 26. PORTLAND, OR

Matt is still taking it easy on his knee and I'm unable to roust the teen so I head out solo. I love Sunday morning runs—lots of other runners, bicyclists, dog walkers, people heading to the bagel shop, or to pick up the paper. I throw a couple of hills into the routine, which helps to remind me that I'm not in really amazing shape—I'm just in consistently decent shape, and I feel good which is better than a lot of alternatives *and* leaves some room to grow.

DAY 82. MONDAY, JULY 27. PORTLAND, OR

My Dad had a rule about staying with friends or family members for a visit—no more than three nights and two nights is better. The idea is that you always want to end a visit thinking that you would have liked to have had more time together. It is true that each time he would leave us we would wish that it could have been longer…always. I think it was a good rule.

I was thinking about it this morning because when I run daily I'm not leaving it all out there on the track or road. I pretty much end every run feeling like I have more in me, that if I had more time, etc., I could, would, or should go longer. For where I'm at these days, this is the perfect way to end a run—ready for tomorrow. It probably wouldn't inspire any hardcore runners, but it's working for me which is all that really matters, right?

PROGRESS REPORT: 283 more days to make a year of this. That's still as many days as I have run already…plus 201 more! Baby steps, baby.

DAY 83. TUESDAY, JULY 28. PORTLAND, OR

I love pedicures, and I get them frequently from a lovely woman I have gotten to know. A few months ago I sat down for one and overheard the woman next to me asking her pedicurist not to scrub the bottom of her feet. "I'm a runner," she said, as if this made sense to the pedicurist. Naturally, I had to ask. We talked about how as we get older the fat pads on the bottom of our feet seem to thin out. For some people it can feel like walking on bone. I periodically have these issues and took a clue from this fellow runner.

You see, normally they scrub the heck out of my feet until they are baby soft all over, including the bottoms. When I was a kid this would have been completely undesirable; in the summertime you were always looking to "toughen up" your feet so you could comfortably walk barefoot. Sadly, I no longer spend long hours barefoot outdoors, but I can still appreciate the sentiment, so I decided to try the no scrub routine. I haven't scrubbed the bottoms of my feet relentlessly since then, and I do notice a difference both in the way that my feet feel on the bottom—more like feet and less like a baby's butt—and in less sensitivity as I've been doing more of my mileage on the pavement than at the track. I think there's something to this obscure idea!

TIP: Don't scrub the bottoms of your feet off in a pedicure. You might need all of your feet to run!

DAY 84. WEDNESDAY, JULY 29. PORTLAND, OR

Another stretch of 100 degree days as far as the iPhone weather app can see, but the early morning is super pleasant. I've thrown stairs and/or hills into my runs since I started running solo again last week (Matt is still nursing his knee). I kind of enjoy the hills but the stairs…I look forward to the day when I am bounding up them instead of what feels like dragging my sorry ass.

DAY 85. THURSDAY, JULY 30. PORTLAND, OR

It's warm and sunny in the early morning. I cross paths with several groups of runners and hear the words "one hundred and four" multiple times. It is forecast to hit 104 degrees today—which is a big deal around here, and everyone, it seems, is up and at 'em early outside. I've been adding a bit of mileage over the last few days and do notice that each time I add an additional mile that I really need to be mindful of planning for the additional time it takes so I can weave that in to my schedule more thoughtfully.

TIP: As the mileage sneaks up on you, be sure to plan for some additional time to get the miles in—lest you be showing up for that important meeting without that much-needed shower!

I also need to be mindful of the road. This morning I stepped into a pothole that gave my foot and ankle a little twist—not so much to derail me, but making me sensitive to the fact that a little misstep can cause all kinds of grief.

Today's message: Mind your mileage and mind the road!

DAY 86. FRIDAY, JULY 31. HOT, HOT, HOT. PORTLAND, OR

One hundred and sixty-one. That's how many steps are in the staircase that I've been hitting during my morning adventures. According to *The Portland Stairs Book*, Portland is home to 196 of these public stairways, many of them hidden and built way back when, used as main thoroughfares until the streets were created.

I always run up to the start with such vigor but about a quarter of the way up my pace is slowing and about 80% of the way I'm ready to beg for mercy. I see a personal trainer punishing his trainee on the stairs this morning and lots of others do their daily penance here too.

I change up my route this morning after the stairs and end up in a section of neighborhood where every street I turn on is made of the old concrete with chunks of rock throughout. That asphalt stuff is merciless on your feet and body (blacktop, if I have to do pavement, is my running road of choice). I won't be heading this way again, but...I will take to the stairs again and soon. I'm going to just keep telling myself how much I like a challenge, and that experiencing a little piece of Portland history is the icing on top.

DAY 87. SATURDAY, AUGUST 1. HOT, HOT, HOTTER. PORTLAND, OR

Today I am grateful for our usually clean air. There was wild-fire smoke on the breeze this morning and my lungs have been irritably protesting for the last hour since I've returned from my run. There was some nutbar on the road today who seemed to be following me on his bike and when I got to the stairs actually grabbed his bike and started running up along with me (and no, this did not appear to be a Cyclocross kind of challenge) so I ran extra hard up the stairs—feeling like I'm gaining some strength but apparently taxing my lungs. Other than that, I'm feeling great; strong in my body and strong in my commitment.

DAY 88. SUNDAY, AUGUST 2. HOT AGAIN. PORTLAND, OR

I probably didn't need that last mojito last night but it was warm and beautiful out as we watched a movie in the back-yard with friends, and they were going down easy.

In the days before this running challenge I probably would have taken a Sunday after a night of partying as a day off, but getting out for a nice easy run, even with a little fuzz in the head, is truly no big deal.

TIP: It's been said that running is an excellent way to move the aftereffects of a party through the system!

DAY 89. MONDAY, AUGUST 3. PLEASANT PORTLAND, OR

It's cooling down a bit and even in the early morning you notice the difference—and it feels good. Matt joins me today for the first time in more than a week. We take it easy and then he has to stop. It's so hard when you have an injury and you just want to get back into it. It feels so good to start again that you go until it hurts instead of stopping before you get to that point.

I notice that I run differently when I'm alone—I really listen to the familiar rhythm of my breath and keep coming back to that in a meditative kind of way. Running with others is more social and fun. Both are good, as is a mix of the two.

DAY 90. TUESDAY, AUGUST 4. PORTLAND, OR

I bumped into a friend on my run this morning and she said, "So, running is all the exercise you need and get." I thought it was a funny assumption. On some days, it *is* the only exercise I get. On other days, there's more: yoga, a hike, bike ride, swimming or dancing in the summer, skiing, and other sports in the colder months. It's true that on some days a quick run is all I get. Mostly, I try to weave in movement wherever I can. Yesterday, I ran in the morning. I walked home from my office, and we took our dinner to Mt. Tabor Park (a popular inactive volcano in Portland, home to many trees and trails) and hiked the park afterwards. I've only been in the elevator in my office building when I've been carrying boxes, and I take the dogs out, even for very short walks, every day that I'm home. Running may be the only time in the day when my heart rate is elevated and I'm sweating—or it may not. At least on those days, I know I will have had that experience. Clearly, there's no one size-fits-all here, but this is what is working for me, right now.

In other news, we dropped Shea off for running camp this morning and find ourselves wishing we could go too, not so much in that "we're going to miss our kid while he's away" kind of way but in a "that's a great way to spend a week, I wish I could do that too" kind of way. I suppose it's never too late!

DAY 91. WEDNESDAY, AUGUST 5. PORTLAND, OR

My run starts with those wicked stairs and then moves into a slow, somewhat labored pace. Sometimes it's straightforward to pinpoint the things that make for an optimal run—rest, hydration, what I've been eating and when, the weather, the course, how many miles I ran the day before...Today is more labored than usual because of some perfect storm of influences. Luckily, I am not out to set any pace records, just out to do my thing and do it consistently.

Speaking of consistency, with yesterday marking 90 days, I checked in on the US Running Streak Association's Facebook page. There were people posting with hundreds, even thousands of days. Wow. Hats off to them! 90 days and I am just a baby taking my first steps.

DAY 92. THURSDAY, AUGUST 6. PORTLAND, OR

En route to Dallas today and sandwiched in the middle seat between my daughter and a man who snorts loudly each time he falls asleep and his head drops back, making us giggle. As I sit here my butt is aching. I so long to get up and stretch and move around like we used to be able to do, but they've gotten so strict about it these days. Today, in particular, I'm extra grateful to have gotten in a run before taking off so that my butt doesn't actually turn into the pancake it feels like right about now.

DAY 93. FRIDAY, AUGUST 7. GRANBURY, TX

There's a scene in the movie *Desert Runners* about long distance runners competing in a grueling (and I mean grueling!) distance race across some of the most inhospitable places in the world when two of the women runners take hands and shuffle along together, holding on to each other for moral support and dear life. Their shuffling comes to mind this morning as I run here. Even at 7:00 a.m. Texas time, the temperature is already 82 degrees, and it feels even warmer. It's predicted to be 110 degrees here today with the heat index (whatever that means—it just says "unbearably hot" to me). I feel like I am moving through molasses, my pace even slower than runs at home when I include stairs. Still, mourning doves, dragonflies, and hummingbirds are a wonderful distraction and when it is done it is done! Phew.

DAY 94. SATURDAY, AUGUST 8. GRANBURY, TX

Up and at 'em earlier to escape some of the heat. It's only a few degrees cooler at this time than yesterday's run, and perhaps I've acclimatized a bit, but it's easier and more enjoyable—and I add just a bit more distance into the mix. The rest of a long day packed with family and activities, I am energized and happy. A great start for the day.

My list of running related movies that I would like to see is way longer than the list of those that I have seen. So much to look forward to! Here are some that I enjoyed this year:

Prefontaine. Pre is a legend to so many and particularly to those of us who live or have lived in Eugene, Oregon. Jared Leto is really compelling as Pre. There are other movies about Pre, *Without Limits* and *Fire on the Track,* that I'd like to see too.

Four Minute Mile: I enjoyed watching this one with my kids, about a high school runner dealing with his unstable inner-city life. It's a movie where running is front and center, and it sparked great family conversations too.

Forrest Gump: I rewatched this movie with my family this year and was reminded of how much of it is taken up by running and by how much we all loved it together. Run, Forrest, run!

The Barkley Marathons: *The Race that Eats its Young*: If you have to ask, you won't understand. Thanks to this movie I spent an entire weekend hitting refresh on my Twitter feed to stay on top of updates from Tennessee and to cheer everyone on!

Desert Runners: Documentary following a group of runners attempting to run 1000km on four different continents in the "driest, windiest, hottest and coldest" places on earth. Wow. Just wow.

Unstoppable: The story of streak runner Robert Raven Kraft who has clocked more than 100k miles during his 40-plus year streak. Perhaps most remarkable to me is not his incredible and uninterrupted streak but the fact that he has run every single day in the same place all of these years. Go, Raven, go!

There are a bunch of running-related YouTube channels I subscribe to now. I've spent many an hour and enjoyed everything I've seen by Billy Yang and Ginger Runner, ultra runners themselves who weave storytelling and adventure and leave me entirely inspired.

Clearly, I'm not the only one who feels this way. Films of this ilk even have their own place now at the traveling *Trail Running Film Festival*.

DAY 95. SUNDAY, AUGUST 9. GRANBURY, TX

I see my sister during my cool down. She is just returning from her daily walk and, inspired by our conversation about the mile-a-day challenge yesterday, she added a mile of running into her usual walk. We talk about the challenges of working full-time and parenting and fitting in a daily run that doesn't interfere with sleep on either side of the day. It's fun to walk and talk together, and we plan to do it again tomorrow.

DAY 96. MONDAY, AUGUST 10. GRANBURY, TX

A run and long walk with my sister. Running at conversational pace and walking too provide a great platform for long, uninterrupted conversation. It's so enjoyable to be able to connect this way! Only wishing I could do this more often.

DAY 97. TUESDAY, AUGUST 11. PORTLAND, OR

Hello, nice, cool, green park to frolic in on my early morning run—about 25 degrees cooler than yesterday's run at this time in Texas! Appreciating running in different climates and vistas to mix it up.

Someone asked me this morning about my favorite little running accessory—my Amphipod. Picture a fanny pack with a miniature pocket instead, big enough for my phone, ID, cash, and maybe a key. I've tried the armband things and I guess my biceps just aren't large enough to keep it on my arm without bouncing around...yet! The Amphipod is light, worn around my hips, and as minimalist as they come. They also make hydration belt versions with little water bottles. Every member of our family has one, and I never run without it. I start the running app on my phone at the beginning of each run, tuck it in and off I go. Highly recommended especially for races when you need a little cash or a gel or a subway ticket!

DAY 98. WEDNESDAY, AUGUST 12. PORTLAND, OR

I had plenty of time to get up and out the door this morning for my run but instead took it leisurely, reading the paper online and responding to e-mail. Before I knew it, the window of time was closing before my first meeting. This used to happen to me all the time. I'd answer just one more e-mail and then I'd lose the time and opportunity to get out the door. Today I got out the door, but barely, which reminds me how tenuous this all is. There's a reason Alcoholics Anonymous uses the "One day at a time" slogan. Never take it for granted and keep the discipline wheels greased!

DAY 99. THURSDAY, AUGUST 13. PORTLAND, OR

My feet and calf muscles are a little achy this morning, likely not due to a run, but maybe from biking to work or some other activity. It gets me thinking about the aches and pains that runners endure, and then I see a friend that's in training for the Portland Marathon. He has run many a marathon and triathlon and all manner of races and tells me about his aches and pains, and how we endure what we do. Mine are certainly nothing compared to his! I'm not much of a "no pain, no gain" girl. I want to stay healthy so I can maintain being active as long as feasible. That is what I am training for!

DAY 100. FRIDAY, AUGUST 14. PORTLAND, OR

When a person trains once, nothing happens.
When a person forces himself to do a thing a hundred
or a thousand times, then he certainly has developed
in more ways than physical.
—Emil Zatopek, Olympic Gold Medalist

I see my friend who is training for the marathon again this morning. His cool down walk is longer than my run today!

A full day today with lots of meetings in between games at my daughter's soccer tournament. My morning runs were short this week, but there they were. While my mileage pales in comparison to most—many people on a streak have minimum mileage for their days set at 5k and higher—I am going to give myself a pat on the back today for sticking with this long enough to hit a the nice round number of one.hundred. days. today!

PROGRESS REPORT: I am beginning to see why so many people get on this streak and then just don't stop!

DAY 101. SATURDAY, AUGUST 15. PORTLAND, OR

I take the dogs with me on my jaunt around the park. A half-mile in, one of them stops to take a doggie dump so after I restart my mile I'm running with a swinging bag of poop in my hand—whee!

As we round the bend above the track we come upon two full-on games of Muggle Quidditch; you know, an adaptation of the game played by wizards and witches on flying broomsticks in the *Harry Potter* series. Yep, grown men and women running with a broomstick between their legs, trying to catch and pass a ball with one hand and send it through the ring-shaped goals on poles on the ends of the field. These folks looked serious and awesome, doing their part to keep Portland weird.

DAY 102. SUNDAY, AUGUST 16. PORTLAND, OR

Matt is back in town and his knee is more tweaked than previously. I miss our running time together, but I'm still feeling pretty pumped to have passed the 100-day mark with no intention of slowing down. Nice and easy run to and around the track this morning.

DAY 103. MONDAY, AUGUST 17. PORTLAND, OR

A jam-packed morning, I want to make it a quick one. I realize I must have paused the mileage on my phone because some time later it still says the same thing! I want to make it legit so I start it over again to make up the mileage. My super quick run will not be as quick as I'd imagined but...it is a stunning morning, so there's that too.

TIP: There are few better ways to start a week out right than with a Monday morning run. Bring it on, week!

DAY 104. TUESDAY, AUGUST 18. PORTLAND, OR

I can tell that Matt is really missing getting out there. Running is just such a good, efficient workout for busy lives. It's hard when injury waylays one part of a team. I miss having a running partner too; I know my distances would be longer and my pace probably faster. Perhaps it's time to consider alternatives...

At the park this morning there are all manner of high school teams having early morning tryouts: soccer, lacrosse, and more. Loving seeing the incoming freshmen getting themselves lined up for high school success!

DAY 105. WEDNESDAY, AUGUST 19. PORTLAND, OR

I run on the track this morning while Ella Donaghu, the Oregon women's high school record holder in the 1500-meter race, runs in the opposite direction. I get barely a quarter of the loop around the track once when she passes me going the other way. Whoosh! So fast, so strong, serious, determined, graceful, and gorgeous! You go, girl! Your future is so bright and your present looks pretty amazing too!

DAY 106. THURSDAY, AUGUST 20. PORTLAND, OR

There are a coach and a woman doing some serious training on the track this morning. She's running across the field on her hands and feet, running sprints around the track followed by laps where she just runs on her tiptoes, etc, etc. She's working hard, training. By contrast, I suppose I am not so much of a runner as a jogger. At least that's how it feels today. I'm not training for anything in particular. I have no other goal than to get out every day, to be consistent, to keep myself in optimal health and to enjoy myself. I watch others who are training like that and think that now is not my time for that, but it may come again.

DAY 107. FRIDAY, AUGUST 21. PORTLAND, OR

We went to a parent meeting for the fall high school cross-country team last night. It's a no-cut team, meaning anyone who wants to join can—no tryouts. It doesn't mean they can just show up occasionally or slack off. They have to be committed, but they don't have to be the fastest or the best. As a result not only is it the largest sports team in the school, it's the largest cross-country team in the state! The positive reinforcement and focus not on winning—though they love to win too—engenders continual improvement and continual striving to make yourself better.

I can remember when I was training for the marathon how thrilling it was to come home from a training run and say, "I ran farther today than I've ever run." And to say that time after time as we made our way to the big distance.

TIP: You can learn so much by tracking your distance and pace over time, watching how they fluctuate and unlocking the recipe for how and why.

Very excited that my kid gets to be part of something so positive, meaningful, and confidence and growth building. As a parent, I'm glad I get to be part of it, too.

My run this morning is a little longer and a little faster than I've been putting in. I think some of this positivity and inspiration is rubbing off on me too!

DAY 108. SATURDAY, AUGUST 22. PORTLAND, OR

The smoke in the air from the wildfires in Oregon and Washington is doing little to discourage all the active folks this morning. In the park I see fitness boot camp, Tai Chi on the basketball court, a half field football team practice, a soccer team scrimmage on the other side with lots of spectators, a mommy and baby fitness class in the grass, dogs all over the dog park, sprinters on the track…This is the last weekend before school begins and it is all starting to happen.

DAY 109. SUNDAY, AUGUST 23. PORTLAND, OR

The smoke got pretty bad yesterday afternoon. It was like a strange and eerie ghost town with people being encouraged to stay indoors. It seemed to shift all day long as the breeze would come and go, and I worried about whether it would be wise to run outdoors—fully recognizing that my little inconvenience was nothing compared to the folks dealing with the situation from closer range.

Fortunately, this morning it doesn't look or feel too bad. Still, I want to err on the side of caution so I run a slow single mile that doesn't get me breathing too hard and call it good. In some ways, it's harder to run slow like that, but for me, for today, it's the right thing to do.

DAY 110. MONDAY, AUGUST 24. PORTLAND, OR

We did a 24-hour backpacking trip on Mt. Hood over last night. My legs felt strong and my body up to task. But, while I covered a lot of ground this last day, none of it was running pace. So…after I've gotten the trail dust off myself and my stuff, it's out the door with my tired bones. Shea missed Cross Country (XC) practice this morning since we were out of town so he runs with me. We are both slow and a little sore. It's a bit like running through molasses, but it's not a huge deal to run a couple of miles. He's kept up his training routine, and I've kept up my consistency.

DAY 111. TUESDAY, AUGUST 25. PORTLAND, OR

I'm annoying myself this morning with so many reasons why I don't feel like running—I'm too busy, too tired, too sore,

I just got my period, blah, blah…I love how so many runners on the US Running Streak Facebook page use the phrase *Thank God I got to run today*! And, so I turn my attitude around by deciding to turn the run into a thankfulness run.

TIP: When you're just not feeling it, get out there anyway and use the run as an opportunity to express your gratitude for running…for anything. Just get out of your head and onto your feet! Be thankful you got to run today.

There are so many reasons to be grateful to just get out the door and I am reminding myself of them as my feet hit the pavement. I'm also thinking about how one of Shea's XC coaches told the parents that the kids aren't always going to like their coaches as they are spurred on to become better runners. I might not always like getting out the door, but so what?! As I walk home on my cool down run I feel like my entire day has turned around. Thank God, I got to run today!

DAY 112. WEDNESDAY, AUGUST 26. PORTLAND, OR

I'm less of a whiner this morning but I still whine. Tomorrow is the first day of school so I attempt to get the kids out of bed at the time they'll need to be up and at 'em tomorrow. I've added a level of activity to my morning that made it more challenging to get out the door to get the run in, and this is only going to amplify as we get into the school year. Ack—I'm still whining! But…I go out there and I do it. And a giant, woolly dog runs across the field in the park and jumps on me just to make it memorable.

DAY 113. THURSDAY, AUGUST 27. PORTLAND, OR

First day of school and I have an early morning meeting. I am up, but the morning is getting away from me as we prepare for this big day. I am dressed and ready to run but about to throw in the towel—this just isn't going to work—when I realize what a bad precedent I would set for myself if I put this run off because school is now back in session and the mornings are more compressed. So…I bang out just a hair more than a mile, shorten the cool down, skip the stretch, and take the world's fastest shower. I did it, I did it, and now it is done. 113 days. Woot woot!

DAY 114. FRIDAY, AUGUST 28. PORTLAND, OR

Shea had his first high school XC meet last night. I really loved the camaraderie, not just among his teammates but among *all* of the teams. Like at a marathon or other road race the spectators are cheering for ALL the runners. I heard things from our coach like: "Run like the wind!" and "You're beautiful!" It flies in distinct contrast to our weekends spent on the sidelines of another sport chasing a black-and-white ball where the kids are challenged to be more assertive, aggressive even, to "get 'em, get 'em!" and where the kids sometimes cry when they are defeated and the parents talk smack about the other team coaches, parents, or players.

Running is all about bettering ourselves—as runners and as people.

My neighbor is on the track this morning, running 30-20-10 intervals. I may need to try that to add a little variety and strengthening into my routine. For now, I'll be happy that I'm bettering myself, one running streak day at a time.

DAY 115. SATURDAY, AUGUST 29. PORTLAND, OR

I have an early morning get together with a colleague over tea and run to the café. I can do this because it's a casual get-together, and I love the efficiency of it all. Afterwards, I decide to run back home as well, since it's faster than walking. Boom!

TIP: Instead of driving, run to a meeting or the post office or to your office—especially if a shower awaits you on the other end!

DAY 116. SUNDAY, AUGUST 30. PORTLAND, OR

Perhaps inspired both by my neighbor running intervals the other day and all the great coaching my son is getting on his XC team, I run some intervals on the track today. Running this way really illustrates how little I am pushing myself when I run. This whole thing started out as an experiment just to see if I could get out there consistently and I am doing that, but now I'm inspired to do more.

When I check my MapMyRun afterwards I see I've logged the fastest miles I've logged in years. I'm proud of my faster pace and yet reminded that the pace I ran at today was exactly my training pace when I was training for a marathon many years ago—in other words, I'm getting faster, but I'm still not that fast!

DAY 117. MONDAY, AUGUST 31. PORTLAND, OR

I decide to run more intervals this morning. I start slower than yesterday because Matt is back out here with me, but even a couple of laps with intervals thrown in have big impact on my overall pace.

Imagining what I could do with my running and in so many other areas of my life if I just kicked it a little harder each time. Hmmmm…

DAY 118. TUESDAY, SEPTEMBER 1. PORTLAND, OR

Matt is out here with me again. He doesn't run the full distance, but it's good to have him back. I run some more intervals on the track—at least I think they're intervals. I'm just throwing variations on sprints of 30, 20, or 10 seconds into my laps as I run around the track, and it is something! I'm shaving time off of my total mileage and that feels great. Perhaps I'll get all geeky about this stuff and start really working it. Until then, another day, another (faster) run.

DAY 119. WEDNESDAY, SEPTEMBER 2. PORTLAND, OR

I spent time today going back through all of my MapMyRun times for the last few months. Ordinarily it's more important to me to just get out there, but I'm starting to really tune into my times. I love the feeling of seeing myself get faster. I haven't added much distance but my times are starting to get back to a zone they haven't been in for a number of years. I'm not going for any records here, but, damn, it feels good!

Honestly, I think the deeper breathing is bringing more oxygen to my cognitive brain. Running just seems to help me think better.

DAY 120. THURSDAY, SEPTEMBER 3. PORTLAND, OR

The kids are a week into the school year, and our new routine is underway. So far, I've been able to carve out the time for a quick run each morning before diving into the big routine of the work and family day.

The weather this morning is the coolest it has been for some time—but I'm not quite ready to say goodbye to summer just yet. I love the warm weather and…at the same time am also praying for a better snow season on the mountain this year than last!

DAY 121. FRIDAY, SEPTEMBER 4. PORTLAND, OR

Solo parenting plus early meetings make the morning extra compressed. I don't get out to run until about three hours after my usual morning time. I haven't eaten yet as I like to do my early runs on an empty stomach, but I have had some caffeine—so I head out, hungry and wired and cold from both the cooler temperatures outside and my own lack of fuel. In the interest of time I keep it just under two miles, but as I run I swear they are some of the fastest miles I've been running in forever and that I'm certainly faster today than I was yesterday. It turned out my split time was just one second faster than the day before though I had thought I was *much* faster. Still, these were faster times than I'd been running a week, month, year ago. I'll take it—though I don't recommend running on (almost) empty.

DAY 122. SATURDAY, SEPTEMBER 5. PORTLAND, OR

I lag getting out the door but I know I'm not going to not go. That isn't an option any longer. I breathe heavier on this run than I usually do—meaning I am pushing myself just a little harder, and it feels...good!

DAY 123. SUNDAY, SEPTEMBER 6. PORTLAND, OR

PROGRESS REPORT: Fastest 5k I've run in years!

Might have been faster if I hadn't been drinking wine last night! But, no complaints here; I've earned my Sunday brunch.

DAY 124. LABOR DAY, MONDAY, SEPTEMBER 7. PORTLAND, OR

I drank more wine last night than I had the night before and outside the temperature has dropped. I'm enjoying the luxury of a long weekend at home by reading in bed, having pulled out my flannel pajamas for the first time since last winter. Wouldn't it be nice just to stay here in bed?! Once upon a time I would have done just that, but I think for a minute about what it would feel like to break my streak—especially just so I could just lounge around for a while, and...I get my butt out of bed and out the door. While it is the slowest and shortest run of the week I'm surprised that it doesn't turn out to be as slow as I'd imagined. Then, I come back and put my pajamas back on! Aaaaah.

DAY 125. TUESDAY, SEPTEMBER 8. PORTLAND, OR

Quick run with Matt before jumping into a shortened week with both feet. It's great to have a running buddy again, though, of course, I'm concerned for his knees. We keep a nice pace. It feels good, and I would like to run longer which is always a good way to end, like the short staying houseguest you wish wasn't leaving so soon!

DAY 126. WEDNESDAY, SEPTEMBER 9. PORTLAND, OR

Today, my lungs cannot keep up with my legs. My first mile is steady and at a standard pace for me. The second turns out to be significantly faster, though I don't realize how much faster until I check my splits on my MapMyRun afterwards. I thought I'd kept pace with yesterday's Mile Two but was clearly well beyond. Not a bad thing, but I think getting the hang of this even pacing[3] thing is not as intuitive as I had imagined!

DAY 127. THURSDAY, SEPTEMBER 10. PORTLAND, OR

I went to a XC meet last night to watch Shea run. I love the way he gets encouraged and coached and for the multiple ways the parents, coaches, and kids are supportive not only of their own teams but of each other. I want to be on a cross-country team! I wonder if they have them for old folks like me.

I know my runs help me stay grounded and sharp for the super compressed days I have on my plate right now. Thank God, I get to run!

---

[3]   Even pacing: pacing yourself at the same time regardless of the terrain when you train (i.e., it's harder and slower to run uphill than downhill).

DAY 128. FRIDAY, SEPTEMBER 11. PORTLAND, OR

Short, speedy and sweet run first thing in the morning.

*If I accomplish nothing else today, at least I have
accomplished my run. What are you going to do today?*

DAY 129. SATURDAY, SEPTEMBER 12. PORTLAND, OR

*Remember, the feeling you get from a good run
is far better than the feeling you get
from sitting around wishing you were running.*
—Sarah Condor, Athlete/Author

Sometimes life gets in the way of creating the ideal circumstances for our runs—or for anything, really. We're too hot, too cold, too hungry, too full, too tired, too busy, too whatever....Some runs are more satisfying than others, but cumulatively the whole running experience is amazing, and days like today with the shortest distance and slowest pace of the week are part of what gives it the context to make it so. Just keep running.

TIP: It's not always going to be easy or fun—do it anyway.

DAY 130. SUNDAY, SEPTEMBER 13. PORTLAND, OR

I aimed to create more time for a longer run at least one day this weekend, but it's not what happened. Today the run is not perfect, not long...but, I'm reminded of a Haitian proverb—little by little a bird builds its nest.

DAY 131. MONDAY, SEPTEMBER 14. PORTLAND, OR

It is significantly darker out there first thing this morning, and there are trees whose colors are beginning to change. Running outdoors year-round really gets you in tune with noticing things in your environment. I feel more connected to the cycle of the seasons

DAY 132. TUESDAY, SEPTEMBER 15. PORTLAND, OR

I see the most beautiful sunrise from the track this morning! It's an amazing reward.

DAY 133. WEDNESDAY, SEPTEMBER 16. PORTLAND, OR

Today I am feeling thankful for all the folks who post on the US Running Streak Association Facebook page. What an inspiring group of folks who support and cheer each other on. I love the spirit of this sport! I can always know that anyone who has a long streak has, at one time, been in exactly the same place that I've been.

PROGRESS REPORT: Fastest run of the month—BOOM!

DAY 134. THURSDAY, SEPTEMBER 17. PORTLAND, OR

Heavy rain this morning. We need it so badly but it is dark and wet. When it's somewhat cold and rainy I struggle with what to wear. It's impossible for your feet not to be drenched, and then there's that dance between wearing rain gear (at least on the top half) that makes you sweatier than you already are or forgoing it and getting wet, cold and immune compromised.

But, allow me to stop with the first world problem agenda long enough to express how uplifted I was by yesterday's experience volunteering in the chute (the finish line area runners funnel through when completing their race) at a high school XC meet. There were coed novice races, JV men and women, and Varsity men and women, and they *all* rule!

So...the finish line is an intense place! It was amazing the number of people—young men and women alike—who burst into spontaneous tears after their race, people who had just left it all out there. I know that particular overwhelming emotion almost always hits me on the finish line. Then, there were the fierce battles to the finish; runners sprinting side by side so they could rank just one number higher than the other finishers. There was the pack of three that pushed so hard at the end that one of them flew into the stanchions on the side and knocked the whole row over. There were lots of finishers who looked like they were going to pass out, a couple we kind of ushered/carried to the end, and one poor kid who barfed after the end. It's hard to imagine anything much worse than barfing repeatedly in front of tons of spectators and teammates, but this kid really took it in stride and I saw his thumbs up not long afterwards.

> *The pleasure of running is rather like that*
> *of wearing a fur coat in Texas in August:*
> *the true joy comes in being able*
> *to take the damn thing off.*
> —Joseph Epstein

So many stories of resilience...the young woman who took first place in the varsity race continued to do speed workouts on the track for the remainder of the event. There seemed to be no doubt that the hard work she was willing to put in was paying off. Then, there was the kid who came in last in the Varsity guys' event—a full five minutes after the last finisher before him. I'd seen this kid at a race a couple of weeks ago, and when I saw his results online I was delighted to see that he'd shaved a full minute off of his last best time. Go, kid, go!

And, finally, there was the runner who crossed the finish line and grabbed my hand. I thought he might need help like some of the others did, but he just shook my hand and said through his panting, "Thanks for volunteering!" How's that for an example of the new generation?!

I am so inspired by these amazing young people and their coaches who work so hard and support each other so beautifully!

PROGRESS REPORT: Slowest run of the month. That's what I get for bragging yesterday!

DAY 135. FRIDAY, SEPTEMBER 18. PORTLAND, OR

I throw in the big staircase today. Stairs are a lot of effort to cover a little bit of distance, but the rest of the run is nice and easy, just the way I'm feeling.

I thought yesterday was the slowest day of the month—well, I guess it was…until today! Thanks, stairs.

DAY 136. SATURDAY, SEPTEMBER 19. TUALATIN, OR

I have 45 minutes between Calliope's warm-up and her soccer game. It's early so I run at the soccer park. The course is hilly and cement and short so I run around the neighborhood around the park too. It's a beautiful morning to be doing just about anything outdoors. I run past garage sales, up and down cul-de-sacs and around a loop twice before I recognize it as such. I'm happy to see another part of town and to mix up my run with features that my usual course doesn't offer.

DAY 137. SUNDAY, SEPTEMBER 20. PORTLAND, OR

The neighborhood runs kind of all blend into one in my mind. I suppose when you do something 100 times or so it's kind of like that! As I sit to write this tonight I have to check MapMyRun to see if the route I'm remembering from this morning is accurate. I was close. And, it was good.

How many other habits could I make so regular as to have a hard time distinguishing one day from another?

DAY 138. MONDAY, SEPTEMBER 21. PORTLAND, OR

This morning is typical of most morning runs. I roll out of bed, put on an old race shirt, a pair of shorts that I bought to run my first marathon almost 10 years ago, my shoes and then I'm out. My hair is still plastered to the side of my head from sleep, and I haven't had any caffeine or brushed my teeth. At the track I see a woman who clearly pays a lot more attention to her run appearance than I. Her hair is perfectly coiffed, a face full of makeup, and a color-coordinated outfit. I don't even look that put together when I put myself together! In the past I might have poked fun (okay, I just did a little) or gloated over lapping her around the track, but today I just celebrate that people of all different shapes and sizes with differing abilities and ambitions, gear and attention to appearances get out there and run. We all have that much in common and probably a whole lot more than we would imagine.

DAY 139. TUESDAY, SEPTEMBER 22. PORTLAND, OR

Compressed days make for short runs, but lots of short runs make for lots of awesomeness. A year ago during this hectic time I was definitely not getting out every day.

PROGRESS REPORT: Loving the streak!

DAY 140. WEDNESDAY, SEPTEMBER 23. PORTLAND, OR

I'm running faster these days so when Matt and I have the opportunity to run together there's less conversation and more heavy breathing. Running...I'm talking about running!

DAY 141. THURSDAY, SEPTEMBER 24. PORTLAND, OR

Yesterday was the first day of fall, but I am still wearing shorts. Another super compressed day, so another shorter run. Short but suh-weet!

DAY 142. FRIDAY, SEPTEMBER 25. PORTLAND, OR

Not much more than a mile today, but done and done.

DAY 143. SATURDAY, SEPTEMBER 26. PORTLAND, OR

Fastest 5k run of the year! Woot, woot!

DAY 144. SUNDAY, SEPTEMBER 27. PORTLAND, OR

Even faster than yesterday! Really?! Yes!

DAY 145. MONDAY, SEPTEMBER 28. PORTLAND, OR

I can still see the supermoon this morning during my run.
That is awesome.

DAY 146. TUESDAY, SEPTEMBER 29. PORTLAND, OR

And another awesome moon in the sky this morning.
Beautiful fall weather, albeit cooler, is making for happy running. These days are just flying by!

DAY 147. WEDNESDAY, SEPTEMBER 30. PORTLAND, OR

Matt was wondering this morning about the probability of
increasing your chance for injury with a streak. I think it's all
about being ultra aware of your body and your limitations
and pushing through them thoughtfully and cautiously—
whether you are streaking or not. As someone who was off
of running for a couple of years because of foot problems
and now as someone on a streak, I can say I am exceedingly
conscientious about approaching it appropriately, and I don't
take it for granted.

Grateful for every day I get to run—like today!

DAY 148. THURSDAY, OCTOBER 1. PORTLAND, OR

I'm seeing the change of seasons through my running. It's been almost five months now!

Last night was another XC meet. A rival team of my son's had a kid on the JV team that is just not what you think of when you think runner. He was big and overweight and slow. And he finished far behind everyone else. But as he did… his team got out there with him to run alongside him, and people lined the track and cheered for him. As he came into the finishing chute the crowd just went nuts. What a brave, strong finish!

Shea said that what he's doing takes way more courage than being the guy at the front of the pack, and there's no doubt in my mind that is true. Go, kid. Thank you for being such a beautiful slice of humanity. And thanks to the coaches willing to work with all levels of athlete and to the teammates and crowds who are part of the awesomeness of all of this.

DAY 149. FRIDAY, OCTOBER 2. PORTLAND, OR

Train, don't strain.
—Arthur Lydiard

I'm feeling a little run down today and want to give my immune system a break so I decide to just run just a bit more than a mile. As I stop, my body is like, "Whaaat? Ready to go more!" which is precisely where it is a good place to stop.

DAY 150. SATURDAY, OCTOBER 3. PORTLAND, OR

Being mindful of taking it easy, I run with the dogs today which is guaranteed to slow me down. They're happy, and I fulfill my intention not to push too hard.

DAY 151. SUNDAY, OCTOBER 4. PORTLAND, OR

A short tempo run at dark o'clock this morning. On travel days like today I'm especially grateful to get my run in before flying and all that sitting.

I had a great talk about running with my cab driver who also has a kid on a XC team. This small world gets smaller all the time.

DAY 152. MONDAY, OCTOBER 5. AUSTIN, TX

I'm taking a beautiful trail run along the Colorado River early this morning. The sunrise over the water is spectacular, and I have the place all to myself save for a group of wildlife photographers in waders in the river and several groups of deer. It feels like an auspicious day to head into a big work event!

DAY 153. TUESDAY, OCTOBER 6. AUSTIN, TX

It is so dark at this hour of the morning that a trail run is out. I run loops around my hotel—anywhere I can find streetlights!

DAY 154. WEDNESDAY, OCTOBER 7. AUSTIN, TX

This morning I discover that the most surefire way to run into people at a conference is to roll out of bed, put on the same stinky workout clothes you wore yesterday, don't brush your teeth, and head to the gym. You will see everyone—and you'll all be in the same "I'm going to kick ass today" club no matter what your hair looks like!

DAY 155. THURSDAY, OCTOBER 8. AUSTIN, TX

We wrap the conference. A smash success. I head out on the trail for a beautiful run, which really brings me back to earth. Now for a big sloppy pizza and some wine!

PROGRESS REPORT: This is the sixth year that I have been part of this multiday work event and the first year I've managed to exercise consistently throughout. That is a welcome shift!

DAY 156. FRIDAY, OCTOBER 9. PORTLAND, OR

An early morning flight and as soon as I landed drove straight to another of Shea's inspiring XC meets (and another PR[4] for him—yay!) then straight home.

We have theater tickets and about 30 minutes to get out the door. We'll probably get home after midnight so now is the time. Matt joins me and we run a pretty slow mile. We get to the theater late but the show starts late, too, and we miss nothing. So glad we got a run in!

DAY 157. SATURDAY, OCTOBER 10. PORTLAND, OR

This morning's run is more of a slog. I'm still depleted from my travels, my calves are sore and I had a huge glass of wine

---

4   Personal Record. Runners striving to top their own best time in an event.

last night, or was it two? But the air feels amazing, and I am on with my day.

DAY 158. SUNDAY, OCTOBER 11. PORTLAND, OR

Even though I would rather sit on the couch with the last three weeks' worth of the Sunday *New York Times* and a cup of tea it is not really hard to get myself out the door for a quick run. My how things have changed!

DAY 159. MONDAY, OCTOBER 12. PORTLAND, OR

It's eerily foggy and beautiful this morning. It feels like it's going to take a few more days to get fully back into the faster and longer swing of things, but I can tell I'm on my way.

DAY 160. TUESDAY, OCTOBER 13. PORTLAND, OR

This week of running was a blur. Nice and fast and short as I get back to my post-event life and routine.

MapMyRun says this run is in my top 25% average pace and yesterday's was top 10%. I'm somewhat surprised but will take this as a nice place to be!

DAY 161. WEDNESDAY, OCTOBER 14. PORTLAND, OR

Today I am back in the top 10% average pace again. Really?!

DAY 162. THURSDAY, OCTOBER 15. PORTLAND, OR

I still bother with runners I call hamburgers.
They're never going to run any record times.
But they can fulfill their own potential.
—Bill Bowerman

And, again in top 10% average pace—a key difference though is that these distances are not much more than streak-saving miles. Even if I'm not comparing apples to apples, it feels good!

DAY 163. FRIDAY, OCTOBER 16. PORTLAND, OR

This was my fastest run yet today. I have to say I am loving being on this curve!

DAY 164. SATURDAY, OCTOBER 17. PORTLAND, OR

I am on a roll in the top 10% again. I'll take it!

DAY 165. SUNDAY, OCTOBER 18. PORTLAND, OR

Keeping the trend by enjoying the short and faster runs. It's also great running weather, which helps…a lot!

DAY 166. MONDAY, OCTOBER 19. PORTLAND, OR

A 5k run is my ideal way to start the week and I did just that this morning. Hooray for weaving enough time into my morning wakeup routine to get 'er done!

DAY 167. TUESDAY, OCTOBER 20. PORTLAND, OR

Today I let my mind wander and I run loops and loops in the park and around the track. Nice pace, easy distance… fun stuff!

DAY 168. WEDNESDAY, OCTOBER 21. PORTLAND, OR

I take the same route as yesterday. Again, it feels like no big deal and I am grateful to be happily enjoying myself!

DAY 169. THURSDAY, OCTOBER 22. PORTLAND, OR

I take the same route but I am much slower today. I suppose all good things must come to an end—only to begin again!

DAY 170. FRIDAY, OCTOBER 23. ROCKAWAY BEACH, OREGON COAST

*Running helps me stay on an even keel and
in an optimistic frame of mind.*
—Bill Clinton

I find two sand dollars as I run along the shore at the beach this morning. The air feels so good. Everything is fresh, and I love making the first footprints of the day in the sand. Ah, Oregon Coast….you are beautiful! What a great place to run!

DAY 171. SATURDAY, OCTOBER 24. ROCKAWAY BEACH, OREGON COAST

I love the way my feet feel landing on the sand. Although I'm wearing my running shoes I can really feel all the parts of my feet as they make contact. There is no excessive pounding, and I feel light on my feet as I make mad dashes up the beach when the waves come in. Running on the beach is one of my happy places. And the long, meandering beachcombing walk on the way back is *awesome*!

DAY 172. SUNDAY, OCTOBER 25. RUN LIKE HELL. PORTLAND, OR

I texted Shea last night and made a typo so Run Like Hell came out like Fun Like Hell, and the name is sticking. Loved this, our third time running this annual festive 5k race today. Shea finished fourth overall and first in his age group. Calliope posted her fastest time ever, inspired by witnessing a few of Shea's recent XC meets I think.

PROGRESS REPORT: I placed in the top five of the women's masters with my fastest time in years. I guess fast girls have great times. Wink.

ALL of us had big fun together. The family that runs together stays together. Go, team!

DAY 173. MONDAY, OCTOBER 26. PORTLAND, OR

I feel so strong on my run this morning. Running up a hill feels like no big deal at all (though the stairs are still a killer!). We have to cut the run short for time, but I feel like I could go quite a bit farther with no problem. Yay for the post-race running boost!

DAY 174. TUESDAY, OCTOBER 27. PORTLAND, OR

I had a hard time getting up for an early run this morning so it will be a short one. The temperature really dropped these last few days, and it is *so* dark in the morning. I think the cold weather makes me run a little faster though!

DAY 175. WEDNESDAY, OCTOBER 28. PORTLAND, OR

A dark and completely rainy run extra early this morning. When I step out the door and see how dark and wet it is I am filled with a dread that evaporates before I'm even out of the driveway. It turns into a fast and fun one. Yay!

DAY 176. THURSDAY, OCTOBER 29. PORTLAND, OR

Nothing remarkable about this run. It's out the door, to the park, round and round the track (which I still find easier on my feet than any other surface). D.o.n.e.

DAY 177. FRIDAY, OCTOBER 30. PORTLAND, OR

Sometimes early morning runs show you things the rest of the world hasn't woken to. I've found wallets, a phone, cash, and more and have been first to see broken car windows or fresh spray paint. On this morning's rainy, windy run through the park there are broken glass and beer cans strewn about, and the XC equipment sheds and bleachers have been vandalized. A sad scenario all the way around. Boo.

You will find stuff when you run! Sometimes it's awesome; sometimes, not so much.

DAY 178. HALLOWEEN, SATURDAY, OCTOBER 31. PORTLAND, OR

Wet, warm, and windy. I rarely drink hard alcohol, but I raised a glass of my Dad's Dutch gin (with tonic) to him last night on what would have been his 57th anniversary with my Mom this week. Though I didn't feel buzzed last night or hungover this morning, I blame that gin and tonic for a run that is on par with others this week but feels harder. Still, it was worth it—both the drink and the run!

DAY 179. SUNDAY, NOVEMBER 1. PORTLAND, OR

How did it get to be November already?!

It rained so hard yesterday and last night that the dog park turned into a literal lake. Usually, early the next morning after Halloween, the streets are filled with the detritus of so much mischief but since Mother Nature kept a lot of people in last night, the only detritus was her own. I love getting up and seeing the world before everyone wakes up. The extra hour of sleep from turning the clocks back didn't hurt either.

DAY 180. MONDAY, NOVEMBER 2. PORTLAND, OR

We caught a bit of the New York Marathon on TV yesterday. Wow—50,000 runners who all qualified at a pretty nice pace. If I were to qualify, I'd need to run a 3:38 or better. When I ran my one and only marathon almost 10 years ago, I did it in 4:09. At that time, I felt I could have done it under four hours, but I'm not sure about 3:38. I am seriously impressed—and inspired. Matt said watching it made him want to run one. That got me pretty excited!

PROGRESS REPORT: Coming up on my six-month milestone. Proud of that too.

DAY 181. TUESDAY, NOVEMBER 3. PORTLAND, OR

Matt has gotten turned on to toe striking in his running. He feels stronger and less injury prone and…it is making him faster. Our first mile usually starts out at a nice conversational pace and then we step it up. Today we hit that first one a full minute faster than our usual pace. This is going to be good!

DAY 182. WEDNESDAY, NOVEMBER 4. PORTLAND, OR

Today is the first morning it's been under 40 degrees in a while, and Matt is still trying on the toe strike for size. Colder weather and toe striking make for a faster run—but this one is shorter because of a compressed schedule and a struggle to rise at the crack of dawn now that it's so darn dark outside in the morning! I loved banging out my run first thing this morning. Now I am ready for what this day has to bring!

DAY 183. THURSDAY, NOVEMBER 5. PORTLAND, OR

Feeling kind of like crappo this morning. I get out of bed late and tell myself I'll just do the minimum mile to get it over with. After the first half-mile I stop feeling so cold and actually feel like I could run a lot more, but I haven't allotted the time. The run really did make me feel better.

TIP: Sometimes when you feel like crap, a run will knock it right out of you.

In addition to feeling better, I'm feeling proud of my freshman who was named the Fastest Frosh at the XC team awards last night with an introduction to the group as the "future of Cross Country!" He and one other freshman teammate even earned their varsity letters. The best part of the night though, was that every single kid was acknowledged. The coaches took their groups to the stage and one by one called the kids up and told a short story about each one— about perseverance, consistency, grit, determination, attitude, and so much more. The parents were all so moved and so grateful for these incredible coaches and the program, wishing there was more of this in the world—both back when we were in high school and now. Feeling so fortunate that my kid who has worked so hard is building his confidence and character both on the track or trail and off.

Oh also…today is halfway to a year. Woot!

DAY 184. FRIDAY, NOVEMBER 6. PORTLAND, OR

Ran solo this morning. Nothing remarkable about this run except for the fact that it's one more brick in a tower built of dedication and consistency—without which the tower would only be so high.

DAY 185. SATURDAY, NOVEMBER 7. PORTLAND, OR

Honestly, it never ceases to amaze me
how much resistance there can be before a run
and how much of a non-issue it becomes
once you just get off your ass.
—Me, This Morning

I was reminded today how much I enjoy getting in my daily run first thing in the morning. Otherwise, like homework or a work deadline, it just hangs over my head until it's done.

This evening I froze my butt off from the sidelines of Calliope's soccer tournament where it's dark and stormy. I was so looking forward to coming home and getting into some warm pajamas and tucking in to a movie with my girl since the boys are out of town. I put some nachos in the oven when we got home, and they smelled so good. My hands were thawing, my mouth was watering, I was about to take a bite…when I realize I hadn't run yet. Dang.

I put on my gear and head out. Since it's dark, cold, and raining, I dress differently than usual and then spend the bulk of the run tugging at my underwear and my sweatpants—both of which are falling down. Still, the mist on my face and the sound of my slow breathing are familiar and make me happy.

DAY 186. SUNDAY, NOVEMBER 8. PORTLAND, OR

I am still cautious with my distance, ever-grateful to be injury free and ever-mindful how small mistakes can cost big—especially when it comes to irritating a neuroma. I hover between 1.5 to 3.5 daily miles. Some days, like today, I would really like to do more.

I run a fun and easy 3.5 while lots of people are up early raking leaves into the street for the first of our annual leaf pickup days. It's kind of festive out here with everyone scrambling before the trucks arrive. I end strong and consider doing more. Like houseguests you are sorry to see leave, this is the perfect time to end it.

DAY 187. MONDAY, NOVEMBER 9. PORTLAND, OR

I drink one cup of caffeine each day—a cup of green tea I have with my breakfast. My morning routine was a little off today (okay, I should have gotten up earlier), and I ended up having my tea *before* my run. Doesn't sound like a big deal, but holy fast run, Batman!

In the first mile I don't miss a beat from the first step. Heading into the second I remember why I usually like to run on an empty stomach, which includes abstaining from food and, apparently, tea. The tea just sits there like a foreign substance my stomach was closing in around. Still...

PROGRESS REPORT: Today's pace was fast enough to land me in my top 10 fastest runs of the last six months. Experience something new each day!

DAY 188. TUESDAY, NOVEMBER 10. PORTLAND, OR

I've been compromising my runs by not getting up with enough time for a longer one. Today I get my butt out the door and Matt joins me and we knock out a quick mile and a half. The streak is still on—longer mileage or not.

DAY 189. WEDNESDAY, NOVEMBER 11. PORTLAND, OR

It's simply that I have to.
—Emil Zatopek, Olympic Gold Medalist

We're remodeling the kitchen in our house, and everything is crazytown. Just making a cup of tea—getting water, finding a place in the bathroom to plug in the teapot, and finding a cup and the tea—is a big effort, not to mention what needs to happen in order to make any food happen. This is the kind of scenario that in the past would have been an excuse for me not to get a run in. I'd think everything was too crazy, too busy, too much something, and I'd use it as an excuse not to get out the door. However, I have upped the ante on what an acceptable excuse might be. My run feels a little ragged and sloppy, but I'm doing it. Streak on!

DAY 190. THURSDAY, NOVEMBER 12. PORTLAND, OR

I think there are a lot of people who owe the success of their streaks to the contributions of others: running partners, inspiration from other streakers, and support from our own family and friends who help us get out there and to keep going. Today I'm thankful for Matt who stays home while I go out so he can take care of meeting with kitchen contractors and helping to get the kids out the door to school.

DAY 191. FRIDAY, NOVEMBER 13. PORTLAND, OR

As I'm leaving the house this morning I think for a fleeting instant about going to go pee before I walk out the door, but I blow it off. I don't have to go that bad, and I just want to get going. Herein lies a lesson.

TIP: When you go out for a run, anything that might be a little thing before you are running can become a big thing when you are out there—a loose shoelace, a tag that rubs the back of your neck, or a semi-full bladder. Do yourself a favor and take care of all of that business before you head out!

BOOKS I READ THIS YEAR

Born to Run: A Hidden Tribe of Superathletes, and the Greatest Race the World Has Never Seen—Christopher McDougall

A true-life adventure so amazing it could be fiction, the story follows the author and a group of American ultra runners to the canyons of Mexico to learn from the ultimate ultra runners, the Tarahumara Indians. Epic.

Finding Ultra: Rejecting Middle Age, Becoming One of the World's Fittest Men and Discovering Myself—Rich Roll

Rich Roll is a plant-powered (vegan) athlete who grabs you with the intimate story of his transformation from seriously out-of-shape guy to endurance athlete extraordinaire, fueled by a super healthy, plant-based diet. Loved it!

Eat & Run: My Unlikely Journey to Ultra Marathon Greatness—Scott Jurek

The author is one of the athletes featured in *Born to Run*, and, like Rich Roll, is a plant-powered monster athlete. Along with his story, Scott includes some of his favorite recipes and reinforced for me that real food is what is going to work for me out on the trail.

How Bad Do You Want it?—Matt Fitzgerald

Good stuff about the physiobiology of what happens during a race and how strong mental fitness helps us push up against our physical edges. Mind over muscles, baby!

> *Racing the Rain*—John L. Parker, Jr.
> This one is fiction and the prequel in a trilogy of novels with running at the forefront. It's the coming of age of an athlete during the 50s and early 60s with plenty of training details woven in to keep the running geeks captivated.

DAY 192. SATURDAY, NOVEMBER 14. PORTLAND, OR

In addition to the rewards that running reaps for me physically, mentally, emotionally and spiritually, today it also rewards me *financially* when I find $20 on the sidewalk. I love it when this happens!

DAY 193. SUNDAY, NOVEMBER 15. PORTLAND, OR

In reading several books lately written by ultra-endurance athletes one thing is evident—part of the race is physical but a big part is mental, drawing upon an amazing well of… *something* that gives these athletes the grit and determination to tough it out when the going is unimaginably intense. Mega ultra-marathoner Rich Roll is an alcoholic. He might be in a deep, dark place—or even dead—without his athletic endeavors. Ultra-endurance legend Scott Jurek endured a childhood that clearly filled his well with experiences that taught him about endurance of many kinds. Yesterday, my daughter's soccer tournament game ended with penalty kicks in overtime. One of the dads kept yelling, "Kick it like you're mad!" I wondered what these girls had to be mad about.

On my run this morning, I'm thinking about how grief has helped me get out to run, but I still don't push too hard. My life is fortunate, things are relatively easy, and I enjoy my runs. They aren't motivated from a gritty place where I'm pushing beyond and drawing upon that well. I keep it comfortable and consistent—yet I wonder what the well that would give me the kind of resilience needed in those situations would look like. Just have to keep digging in, I guess.

When I started this running streak I thought the conditioning would be physical and a bit of mental—mostly to just get out the door—but now I see that to really excel at this there's a whole lot more of the mental to develop and condition. Good thing I like a challenge!

DAY 194. MONDAY, NOVEMBER 16. PORTLAND, OR

On today's run I'm grateful for Matt who stayed home to take care of so many things that were converging at once so that I could go out for a quick one. He's definitely carrying the heavier load today by supporting me to get out. Matt, I'm thinking of you as I huff my way up every one of these stairs!

DAY 195. TUESDAY, NOVEMBER 17. PORTLAND, OR

Feet. Shoes. This is what's on my mind as I run this morning. I'm only out here because I was able to manage a debilitating neuroma years ago, and it is never far from my mind.

Fortunately I don't have to dress super fancy for work every day because, truthfully, otherwise I'd be hosed. I've never been big on high heels or uncomfortable shoes, but I can tell you that as a woman 99.9% of all shoes out there have a toe box that assumes your normal shaped foot tapers into a nice pointy point at the front—which it does not—thereby forcing your toes and metatarsals to squish together and causing a neuroma if you're unlucky.

Sadly, even for the unfashionable like me, there are still just not enough choices that are kind to our feet. So, all summer long you'll find me in Birkenstocks when I'm not running.

Luckily, Birkenstocks have come a long way from Grateful Dead tour days and come in colors and styles that even people who don't care about their feet are wearing. In the colder weather, I struggle. I wear old running shoes as often as possible when I'm not running and UGG boots where I can get away with them. Flats are completely out since they have zero cushioning in them, and my poor feet just can't handle that anymore.

When I have a spell where I have to dress up for days, even with the best of the best of women's shoes with the wider toe box and lower heels, my feet bark like dogs. I don't know how other people manage it, but I have to say that being überconscious about what I put on my feet has been a game changer for me, worth giving up form for function. No turning back.

DAY 196. WEDNESDAY, NOVEMBER 18. PORTLAND, OR

I really shouldn't blame solo parenting while Matt is out of town for not getting a longer run in. The fact is, if I had gotten up when my alarm went off the first time I would have had plenty of time. The mile is good but longer would be better. Good thing there's always tomorrow!

DAY 197. THURSDAY, NOVEMBER 19. PORTLAND, OR

When I first moved to Oregon a number of years ago I gleaned some good advice on how to deal with the perpetually rainy weather. Having come north from California I'm not sure I knew what I was really in for, and these two things helped me through:

1. Plant a garden. Then every time it rains you can be happy and thankful that you don't have to water.
2. Have the right gear. If you have the right gear, then getting out in the elements is no big deal.

I remind myself of that #2 this morning as I put on my shell and head out. No big deal.

TIP: Get the right gear to run in all kind of conditions, and then you have no excuse to not get out the door. It doesn't have to be fancy, just functional.

DAY 198. FRIDAY, NOVEMBER 20. PORTLAND, OR

I moved through a day with call after meeting after call on top of solo parenting. We also still have a crazytown of a house due to the remodel and guests arriving tomorrow. Through all this I keep a smile on my face the whole day and a sharp, clear head. I attribute my daily run to keeping me in top form not only physically but emotionally and mentally, too. Yay for running and doing it consistently!

DAY 199. SATURDAY, NOVEMBER 21. PORTLAND, OR

A perfect run has nothing to do with distance.
It's when your stride feels comfortable.
—Sean Astin

I see ice in a birdbath this morning. Brrr…The kitchen remodel is in full swing and our guests will be arriving. Matt is out of town and my workweek has been super compressed.

I get up before dawn and start making sense of this remodel mess—my goal being to clear enough space in the room and on the table so we can sit and enjoy ourselves and eat together! I can't believe how much there is to do before they arrive and…I still go out and get my run in. I think it's why I am able to take this whole situation in stride and enjoy it.

Note to self: I wonder if the stress reduction effect of running is the origin of the expression "take it in stride!" Hmmm…

DAY 200. SUNDAY, NOVEMBER 22. PORTLAND, OR

Coldest morning yet. It's Sunday so I am able to procrastinate getting out the door hoping it might warm up a bit more. We are just not acclimated to the cold here, and I am a complete wuss when it comes to these things. I seem to wear three times as many clothes as anyone else in the winter. So this morning I bundle up for my run—wearing my long tights for the first time since starting this streak and a hat and polar fleece jacket over my long sleeved running shirt. By the time I hit a mile I am so uncomfortably warm, except for spots on my ankles and neck that are exposed. Geez, I've got to get used to this and ensure I've got the right gear soon to make my cold weather runs more enjoyable! Two hundred days and still a rookie.

DAY 201. MONDAY, NOVEMBER 23. PORTLAND, OR

Brrr....but I warm right up—right up the stairs! It makes my pace so slow, but what a great workout. And thanks to Matt for taking one for the team so I could get out the door when I did.

DAY 202. TUESDAY, NOVEMBER 24. PORTLAND, OR

My thumbtips are so very cold on this otherwise lovely run!

DAY 203. WEDNESDAY, NOVEMBER 25, 2015. PORTLAND, OR

I should add extra mileage to burn up some pre-Thanksgiving celebration calories, but I don't. The road is a bit icy in the shady spots, and frost is covering everything. It's refreshing and beautiful and cold and an awesome way to start the day!

DAY 204. THANKSGIVING, THURSDAY, NOVEMBER 26. THANKFULNESS RUN. PORTLAND, OR

Shea's XC team has this wonderful tradition of a run at a local park on Thanksgiving. It's been happening for 20+ years, and everyone is invited. It's not a race; the idea is to have in mind who or what you are thankful for as you run laps around the park. Today the coach does a lap for his wife and one each for his kids.

We go as a big family and meet more families and friends and the team there. It is a beautiful clear crisp morning—perfect for a run. I can't possibly run as many laps as things that I am thankful for but I do keep people close to my heart in mind as I run and am especially thankful for good health that allows us all to run and for the running community we are surrounded by. I am also thankful for the pumpkin pie I'll dive into shortly!

DAY 205. FRIDAY, NOVEMBER 27. PORTLAND, OR

It's the day after Thanksgiving and more indulging is around the corner. I would have to run really, really far to make up for *all* of the excess but luckily with this running consistency I'm at least keeping it all in balance—and that feels good!

TIP: Do what you need to do to ensure you get your runs in during the holidays. It will make the whole season infinitely more enjoyable.

DAY 206. SATURDAY, NOVEMBER 28. PORTLAND, OR

I let myself sleep in today (a relative term for a parent, as any parent can attest) after hosting a houseful of guests over the Thanksgiving holiday, so I missed getting out in the morning.

It is a beautiful, clear day that feels more like fall than winter. I have a nice, short, easy run carrying the weight of a little more bread, cheese, pie, and other desserts than I might not ordinarily have indulged in. Fortunate to both have the choice to indulge like that and be able to run it off.

DAY 207. SUNDAY, NOVEMBER 29. PORTLAND, OR

I love Sundays when there aren't major family activities planned and I can be more spacious around and during my run. Yay for Sunday rundays!

DAY 208. MONDAY, NOVEMBER 30. PORTLAND, OR

It's so dark and the temperature is in the 20s this morning! As I moan about how cold the tips of my thumbs are on my little jaunt I can't help thinking about how much of running is in the head and about the incredible inconveniences, discomfort, and full out pain that ultra-runners doing mega distances put themselves through. Suddenly my thumbs don't feel quite so cold anymore!

DAY 209. TUESDAY, DECEMBER 1. PORTLAND, OR

A nice quick one through the park and around the track. I'm enjoying the crisp, sunny morning—the last one in the forecast as far as the eye can see. The crappy, cold rain is coming. Until then, though, the clear sky and brisk temperature is a treat. And I am thinking of inventing thumbwarmers—just partial finger warmers for my thumbtips when I run, which for now seem to be the only part of me getting and staying cold on these near winter morning runs!

Warm hands, warm heart: Depending on your weather conditions, keeping your hands warm while running can be tricky. Cold fingers are no fun, but neither are hot sweaty hands. To find your happy place try experimenting with anything from $1 stretchy gloves for milder days to ski mittens when you're aiming to avoid frostbite.

DAY 210. WEDNESDAY, DECEMBER 2. PORTLAND, OR

For the first quarter mile of the run the wind's blowing so strongly that I groan audibly. Thankfully it's either letting up or I'm ceasing to notice it, and the run has turned pleasant. It's so dark in the mornings that I've been waiting until it's lighter and slightly warmer to go out, which compresses my time. Today I promise myself I'll get out earlier tomorrow, even in the dark, just to get more time in because I enjoy it so much.

DAY 211. THURSDAY, DECEMBER 3. PORTLAND, OR

Matt went for a run with Shea the other day and messed up his leg trying to keep up. There's a lesson in there to be sure!

This morning he attempts to head out with me but only gets about an eighth of the way down the block before abandoning ship. It reminds me of my one and only marathon experience. I'd been training with a group and had naturally fallen in with one woman in particular because our paces were similar. When it came to the marathon, we had run the first 18 miles together when she started really slowing down.

We hadn't necessarily made a commitment to run side-by-side for the entirety, and when she said, "Go on without me" as we were heading up a gentle incline, I did. I thought about her for the rest of the marathon. Was she going to make it? Did she drop out? I remember seeing her husband at the side of the route at one point wearing a big question mark on his face when he spotted me without her. As it turned out, she finished about 15 minutes after I did—about two minutes more per mile than I had run at the end. Not insignificant. I also think about two other women we'd trained with who had finished about 15 minutes before me and somehow feel that I could have kept up with them.

In the future, and particularly for a longer race, I'm going to have a game plan in place. I think I'd like to run with someone or a pace group that both matches and pushes me and with a contingency plan that either says we stay together no matter what or we don't. Running and learning.

DAY 212. FRIDAY, DECEMBER 4. PORTLAND, OR

> *Running improves my relationships with my family,*
> *my friends, everyone around me.*
> *And while my running is personal,*
> *it's also something I give.*
> *Running can be given.*
> —Tony Sandoval, MD,
> Winner of the 1980 US Olympic Marathon Trials

Supercharged by my run for a super packed day full of meetings and calls. Runs really do fill up my reserve for days like these!

DAY 213. SATURDAY, DECEMBER 5. PORTLAND, OR

I decided to take a short easy one since we're running the Jingle Bell Run tomorrow. Afterwards we headed out to the Nike XC Invitational High School Meet. The star female runner from Shea's high school team was running, and we wanted to cheer her and the others on. If you've ever been to a XC meet you know that the thing to do is to watch the start and then run across the field, intersecting the course, to see the runners come up in a different part. As soon as you see them pass, you dart across the course to intersect with the runners at a different place, and so on, so you can see how the race is progressing. It was raining and the field was muddy and a bit hilly. I think I got a harder workout running over the course than I did on my actual run this morning! So much for taking it easy.

The race, like all XC races, was inspiring, and Nike did a first class job with beautiful shuttle buses (including booties for our muddy feet on the return trip) for everyone, friendly staffers, a beautifully marked course, sheltered spectator areas, live webcast, jumbo screen, and just overall a first class production. What a great experience for these kids, coaches, and families who all work so hard to support these runners. Well done, Nike, and well done, runners, teams, coaches, families, friends and other supporters!

DAY 214. SUNDAY, DECEMBER 6. JINGLE BELL RUN. DOWNTOWN PORTLAND, OR

It is pouring when I wake up this morning for our fourth running of the Jingle Bell Run 5k. Amazingly, the weather clears up and, in fact, is even sunny by the end of the race despite the forecast having called for 90% chance of rain at that time. I end up as the seventh female finisher, second in my age group, 35th overall, and I cut about 35 seconds per mile off of my time from last year. BUT...I was so frustrated to have had to stop running for precious seconds just after the first mile to let a train and then a bus pass. Argh! I definitely let out a couple of expletives under my breath. I know the police were doing their job, but it is so disheartening to have to abruptly halt and wait. Argh, ack, bleh, darn!

Still, happy with the way the run went with all of us doing great and Shea taking third place overall. Matt was in San Francisco last night, flew in early this morning, and went right from the airport to the race. I think he wins the biggest award of all for that. This has been such a fun way to spend time together, and I loved being home before 10:30 a.m. to enjoy the rest of the day. Yay!

TIP: Running a race early in the morning can make you feel like you have accomplished so much by the time that most people are just rolling out of bed. And you can always go back to bed after the race too!

DAY 215. MONDAY, DECEMBER 7. WASHING AWAY IN PORTLAND, OR

When it rains in Portland in the wintertime it's not terribly cold like it is on the bright, clear days, but it *pours*.

I don't think it stopped raining all night. As I head out in the dark this morning, about a quarter block into it I am ankle deep in a cold puddle. Ack! It's shocking and wakes me right up. It happens again as I make my way to the track.

Amazingly, my feet aren't cold and there are a bunch of people running on the track with their headlamps on. For the rest of the run I focus on the rhythm of my breath and also listen to the squish, squish of sopping socks and shoes. How did you start your day?

DAY 216. TUESDAY, DECEMBER 8. PORTLAND, OR

My running shoes are still wet from yesterday. Oops, my bad. But, the outside air is warm and balmy, and the mist feels good on my face. I'm loving my new water-resistant jacket. (Note: Water-resistant, not waterproof, which just makes you sweat way more than you do already.)

I have a theory that endorphins don't really kick in unless I've run three or more miles. I do get an energetic burst and head clearing from a quick mile or two in the morning, but more mileage seems to give me more of a mellow euphoric feeling for the rest of the day, which I love.

I have the interesting experience of running half my run with Matt today, then half solo. He's running gingerly now so our pace is slow and the time is great for conversational connection. After he heads back, I am much more in tune with my breath and my own thoughts and have a few of what feel like really good ideas. Today, I love the combination of running together then alone.

Here are some ideas to help with your gear post-run:

Save that newspaper. Stuffing newspaper into wet shoes is the best way to dry them out. Replace newspaper as it gets soggy.

Protect your investment. Despite how much this gear gets used, it seems its biggest workout sometimes is in the wash. I've found that washing in cold water and air-drying when possible helps things hold up a lot longer.

DAY 217. WEDNESDAY, DECEMBER 9. PORTLAND, OR

I read an article today citing a study from the Mayo Clinic that found that "running for about 50 minutes each week—or approximately six miles—can protect the body from risk for stroke, arthritis, diabetes, high cholesterol, high blood pressure, and even some cancers." A little bit goes a long way!

When I was running my first hundred days it wasn't often that I ran much more than a mile per day. More distance means more time running, which means earlier starts.

PROGRESS REPORT: In the days from 100 to 200 I averaged two miles per run. Now in my days from 200 to 300 days, I'm averaging three miles. I can see where this is going!

DAY 218. THURSDAY, DECEMBER 10. PORTLAND, OR

For the Jingle Bell Run last Sunday I wore a pair of my holiday sweater knee socks. They just make me smile. For the rest of the week I've followed suit, wearing a pair of fun socks each day. Today I'm wearing a pair of red knee socks with a Corgi dog pattern on them that Calliope gave me for Christmas when she was 10 years old. I consider them my good luck socks, and they remind me not to take myself or anything else too seriously. It's fun to wear the socks where the world can share in their awesomeness today. I think they help me run faster too!

DAY 219. FRIDAY, DECEMBER 11. PORTLAND, OR

More happy socks = more happy running.

I'm a pretty low-tech kind of runner. I don't have a lot of fancy running clothes to muck up, and everything else is pretty basic. That said, I've loved every recent addition to my running stable: new shorts, tights, running bra, jacket, padded socks, race shirts, and my Knuckle Lights.

Next up: A watch and tracking upgrade. Hello, Santa?!

DAY 220. SATURDAY, DECEMBER 12. PORTLAND, OR

I *really* like my weekend morning runs when I'm out the door before the kids wake up and I don't have to rush back for the whirlwind of getting them off to school as I dig in to my workday. Today, we do have to head out for an annual community service project, but we don't have to pack lunches or homework, which make it feel so much more spacious. More spaciousness means more time to run in my happy socks and a 5k to start the day. Having run hills and stairs on all my other runs this week, running a flat route make me feel so fast—like swimming with the current in the river makes me feel like Michael Phelps. Yay!

DAY 221. SUNDAY, DECEMBER 13. PORTLAND, OR

I ran four miles this morning and then made teacher gifts, baked more than 15 dozen cookies, hosted a birthday dinner for my daughter, and did work, homework for my leadership program, housework…a whirlwind of productivity today and I didn't lose any steam until bedtime. I was no doubt energized by my morning run—that thing about the endorphins kicking in after three miles seems to be the ticket. I could get used to this!

DAY 222. MONDAY, DECEMBER 14. PORTLAND, OR

It has snowed more than 40 inches on Mt. Hood in the last 72 hours, and we are going to get in our first ski runs of the year—in between meetings and working. Yay! A mile and a half feels like enough before jumping into this day with both feet…and boots!

DAY 223. TUESDAY, DECEMBER 15. PORTLAND, OR

My schedule, like everyone else's, is ridiculously overfull right now trying to jam in as many meetings as possible before I take off for vacation on top of the holidays, birthdays, choir concerts, white elephant gift swap, high school fundraising art night, teacher gifts, cookie exchange with the neighbors, etc., etc., ad nauseum.

Today is definitely what I would call a streak-saving mile! I get up too late to get my run in, so I text my meeting mate to ask if we can bump it 15 minutes later and jam out that mile!

TIP: Did you know that running a regular mile generally doesn't even burn 100 calories?! If you're like me, you'll need to run a whole lot more than one mile if you want to balance out some Christmas cookies!

DAY 224. WEDNESDAY, DECEMBER 16. PORTLAND, OR

I took a midday break to go skiing again today (shhh…don't tell the boss!). Interestingly, instead of finding that running and skiing in one day tire me out I actually felt energized all the way through the work and the skiing and more work and evening meetings and homework and holiday prep. Feeling good!

Rather than diminishing, doing more physically seems to be expanding my capacity to do all kinds of other things.

DAY 225. THURSDAY, DECEMBER 17. PORTLAND, OR

When I woke up at 5:30 a.m. I thought I'd put my new hot pink Knuckle Lights to good use for a run in the dark. But… it was so dark and it was pouring outside and the cat nuzzled her way under the covers and it was just so cozy…I reset my alarm for 6:00 a.m. but hit the snooze all the way to 7:00 a.m. Ack.

I finally go out for a quick one in the rain, although I should qualify this by saying it isn't really rain at all but rather big, fat, wet ice bombs falling from the sky. Just one landing on my shoe is enough to make my feet wet, and my underwear and jogging bra are soon to follow. Still, instead of a soggy dog, I feel like a badass out here and the combination of the cold weather and a pair of happy socks really do make me pick up the pace. Woot!

DAY 226. FRIDAY, DECEMBER 18. PORTLAND, OR

Runner's World ran an article recently entitled "Why Are Morning Runners So Happy? " A new study suggests that if you hit the road before having breakfast you might be more likely to experience runner's high.

I'm not sure I follow the whole scientific part of the study but I do know that, like today, knocking out a run before I prioritize anything else for the day makes me feel accomplished and happy and I'll take that!

DAY 227. SATURDAY, DECEMBER 19. PORTLAND, OR

Calliope and I were talking about my running streak this morning, and she decided to join me on the run. Happy dance! We run to the track, and then I run some laps backwards while she runs forwards. In case you haven't experienced this sensation before, I feel like I am just flying when I turn back to running forward. What an awesome feeling! My girl doesn't have distance endurance yet but, man, can she sprint! So fun!

DAY 228. SUNDAY, DECEMBER 20. CANCUN, MEXICO

When I was still up at midnight with so much yet to be done before our trip I almost went for a run but couldn't make the time. I ended up getting about an hour and twenty minutes of sleep before we had to get up for our flight.

My butt was so ready to take a break from all of the sitting on our flights. (I know, first world problem, but so much sitting whether you are on a flight or in an office or on your couch is too much sitting. It just doesn't feel good and isn't good for you, and on flights they don't let you get up like they used to. Rant over.)

We meet Matt halfway across the country. He hadn't gone to sleep at all the night before. We meet up with family at our destination, have dinner with plenty of wine, and get situated. Matt and I are like zombies. At a certain point I can feel my cognitive functioning slowing to a standstill.

And…we get a run in just before midnight Cancun time. I don't have connection on my phone so my MapMyRun isn't happening. I set a timer on my phone knowing that if I run for a certain number of minutes I'll be sure to have hit at least a couple of miles, and that's what we do. It's dark, it's humid, we're exhausted but happy. Despite or because of the run before bed, I fall fast asleep as soon as I have showered. A deep, restful sleep. Hello, vacation.

DAY 229. MONDAY, DECEMBER 21. CANCUN, MEXICO

Wow—deep, deep sleep. Matt passes on the run. I head out on the same route as last night. The road is lined with palm trees, birds-of-paradise, hibiscus, and all kinds of vines. Along the way I see numerous enormous iguanas. I pass a couple of other runners. They look about as accustomed to the heat and humidity as I. I run for half an hour and then to the restaurant to meet Matt for breakfast. It's a lovely start to a lovely day with loads more physical activity: ocean swimming, pool swimming, fitness class, beach walking…Aaaah.

DAY 230. TUESDAY, DECEMBER 22. CANCUN, MEXICO

> *There's nothing like running on the beach.*
> *It's a wonderful sensation.*
> —Bill Lawrence

> *I think Bill might have been running on a*
> *different beach than I when he said that.*
> —Me

Matt and I run on the beach this morning, and it is challenging! The sand is white and soft here and the beach has a steep drop-off so the run is on a slant that your feet sink into deeply. The pace is snail-like.

To be clear, though, I am only reporting—not complaining! The view is amazing, the air feels incredible, and it beats running with ice bombs falling from the sky any day. Hooray!

DAY 231. WEDNESDAY, DECEMBER 23. CANCUN, MEXICO

Strong tropical wind—wow! I stick to roads and paths today. The palm trees and my hair are all blowing sideways, and the wind makes an incredible howling. I ate like a bottomless pit last night; between that and the never-ending stream of beachfront mojitos and wine bottles that flow like an infinity pool I am extra grateful to have the consistency of running in my routine here. I am getting plenty of other exercise, jumping waves and body surfing—just getting pummeled for hours—sailing, yoga, and aerobic exercise classes, but my run is my rock and keeps my head on straight. I'm glad I won't be having to pick up where I left off after I get home, but rather just continue. Yes, grateful.

DAYS 232, 233, 234. THURSDAY, FRIDAY, SATURDAY, DECEMBER 24, 25, 26. CANCUN, MEXICO

This may well have been the first time I've ever run on Christmas Eve and Christmas Day. My runs have been at different times over the last few days. Yesterday's was so hot and humid. The day before I ran on the treadmill in the gym, which was also hot and humid—but I got to run next to Shea and we saw fish jumping in the lagoon as we got in our miles. This morning I ran first thing, which is my preferred timing.

Yesterday I read about someone who unintentionally broke their almost two-year streak because they simply forgot to run. I can see how that can happen when you don't get it done first thing and you need to pay extra attention on vacation. Yikes.

PROGRESS REPORT: I've been reflecting on all the days and places of my life since I started this streak. What I didn't know when I began was that through my own efforts and the camaraderie of the US Running Streak Organization I would find another thing in my life that is consistent, rock solid…through all kinds of weather, places, and scenarios I am running every day, and I am so grateful for that.

DAY 235. SUNDAY, DECEMBER 27. CHEMUYIL, MEXICO

I started to leave for this morning's run, but when I stepped out the door of our jungle Airbnb I saw that our hostess had set up a beautiful outdoor breakfast just for us and I felt like it would be rude to delay. The rest of the day was filled with swimming, snorkeling, hiking, sightseeing—an epic adventure day.

By the time we return to the Airbnb it's dark. There are no streetlights here in the jungle; indeed, there really isn't anything you would really call a street either! We notice a soccer stadium near town that is always lit, so we drive there and do loops around the field. It must look funny, but each loop around the field is a quarter mile so round and round we all go. Shea laps me, and Matt and Calliope give him some good competition by sprinting. Love having a vacation adventure with my family, and love running together too!

DAY 236. MONDAY, DECEMBER 28. CHEMUYIL, MEXICO

Perhaps my most unusual run yet, Matt and I run at night by the lights of our iPhones on a rocky, sandy, uneven jungle road. The moon is not yet up, and while the stars are out I dare not take my eyes off of the road in front of me for fear of a misstep. The air is warm and humid, the crickets are chirping, the bats are flapping, and our run is in the books.

DAY 237. TUESDAY, DECEMBER 29. CHEMUYIL, MEXICO

I managed to get my jungle run in first thing this morning. I pass by a turquoise cenote (the natural underground swimming holes the Yucatan peninsula is known for) and colorful birds fly overhead. In my experience, vacation seems to be the time when many people fall out of their practices: exercise, eating well, quiet time for meditation, and so on are all more challenging when on the road.

PROGRESS REPORT: I made it through this 10-day trip without missing a day of running. Yaaaas!

The days when I didn't get it together early enough to run first thing were the most challenging, but it was fun to get it done with the support of my family.

DAY 238. WEDNESDAY, DECEMBER 30. PORTLAND, OR

From the sandy jungle to the icy blacktop—phew. I wait as long as I can to head out this morning but it is still 30 degrees by the time I leave, and the road is icy. I would call this one more of a shuffle than a run, leaping up into the grassy spots along the way to the track to leverage some traction. Not my favorite conditions but…so what?! Run done.

DAY 239. THURSDAY, DECEMBER 31. PORTLAND, OR

Brrr…last run of the year and first run with my new Garmin watch, which I love. (Thanks, Santa!) It's so cool to have my distance, pace and time right there and to feel the ping on my wrist with each mile.

I am so grateful for all of the running this year and am already looking forward to hitting my 365 in the new year. Bring it!

PROGRESS REPORT: Seven states, two countries, one airport, sun and sand, icy rain, glorious fall and spring, tracks, trails, parks and roads, and three 5ks—all PRs (personal records).

DAY 240. NEW YEARS DAY, FRIDAY, JANUARY 1. PORTLAND, OR

Brrrr....Wowee, it's WINDY and cold and sunny and an awesome day to run to start the New Year off right. HAPPY NEW YEAR of running!

As they say...tracking your progress is the key to success, and if "they" say it, then it must be true!

When I first started out, I was tracking my runs via the **MapMy Run** app on my phone. There's a free version, or you can upgrade. I love how it calls out your distance while you're running and saves your run data including pace, distance, time and the GPS map of your run afterwards. I carry my phone with me anyway when I run, so it's convenient enough that way, however, I was finding it frustrating to have to whip out my phone to get it to pause or stop the run.

I've upgraded to a **Garmin Forerunner** watch, and I love it. It buzzes at each mile mark so you don't even have to look at your wrist for that, but if you do you'll also see your pace, time and distance there at the ready. The online saving of the data is really handy, too.

One app I love is **StreakTrackr**. Just enter your start date, and it tracks the number of days in your streak for you so you don't lose, er...track.

Another option for sharing your routes, distance, time and pace is social network **Strava** which connects to your Garmin or other GPS devices to compare and compete with others. I am an aspiring Strava user but I'm not quite there yet.

DAY 241. SATURDAY, JANUARY 2. PORTLAND, OR

A sunny, cold and windy, sub 30 degree 5k to start the day. I am definitely warm now!

DAY 242. SUNDAY, JANUARY 3. PORTLAND, OR

Snow! It's only every handful of years that it snows in Portland and sticks and…today is our day! I love the silence and softness underfoot as I run along. From the sand to the snow in one week. I love it all!

DAY 243. MONDAY, JANUARY 4. PORTLAND, OR

Crunch, crunch, crunch….Usually when I get in a rhythm as I run by myself, I listen to the sound of my breath. We had an ice storm last night and the whole city is like a skating rink. It wasn't until early evening that the roads were thawed enough to brave going out. Because the pavement is too slick, I run in the grass to the park and get in my 5k on the track, but instead of tuning in to my breath, the only thing I can hear is the crunching of the crusty snow underfoot. My pace needs to be slow because it's pretty treacherous. Between the slowness and the crunch I am feeling pretty Zen.

Kudos to **Knuckle Lights** for innovating something that needed to be innovated by taking the bouncing light from my headlamp and putting it in my hands. It makes me feel safe when it's dark, and they're expandable to fit around my fuzzy mittens to boot!

DAY 244. TUESDAY, JANUARY 5. PORTLAND, OR

When Matt suggested waiting until we'd arrived to our destination across the country today to do our run, my response was an emphatic "No way!" I need the run before I'm going to sit on my rump all day in a plane—in fact, I'll need a run on the other end of the journey too!

The kids have another day off of school today because the snow turned to ice and hasn't yet magically disappeared. We gingerly crunch our way uphill to the bank to get some cash for the trip. Matt says it sounds like we have chain link fence stuck to the bottom of our feet! I feel like I am making better decisions on where to place my feet on the ice based upon my shuffle. If I were walking I might space out a bit, but I am all focus, not wanting to fall on my arse. I find myself really appreciating the adventure of it all—and all the adventure that running brings to our lives!

In the midst of regular life, running is the touchstone
that breathes adventure into my soul.
—Kristen Armstrong, Olympic gold medalist

DAY 245. WEDNESDAY, JANUARY 6. DANIA, FL

Sometimes a run is just a streak-saving mile. Today I did just that on the treadmill in our hotel before a breakfast meeting. With the time zone difference I was in the hotel gym by about 4:00 a.m. Portland time on not enough sleep. #firstworldproblems

DAY 246. THURSDAY, JANUARY 7. MSC DIVINA CRUISE SHIP, ATLANTIC OCEAN BETWEEN FLORIDA AND MEXICO

I haven't been this purple in the face since I ran the Eugene Marathon many years ago. I am absolutely hot, sweaty, purple, and nauseated. I never know how to pace myself on a treadmill. It seems they're all calibrated differently, and the distance and pace feel so different than what that distance and pace feel like on the track, road or trail. Also, Matt and I just wanted a glass of wine with dinner last night but it was about the same price to buy a bottle as it was to buy two glasses, and we figured someone might come join us at our table so we could share. But, no one did, so…we drank the whole bottle. With long hours over the last couple of days, lack of sleep and sufficient food, time zone differences, and a rocking boat I am feeling it.

The best part: knocking out three miles and getting 'er done. The hardest part: staying centered on the treadmill as the boat rocks side to side. The worst part: the pumping remixes of songs I never really liked in the first place blasting through the gym speakers. Plus, I smell bad.

Tomorrow, I vow, I will run outside on the upper deck, even if I have to go 'round and 'round and 'round.

DAY 247. FRIDAY, JANUARY 8. COSTA MAYA, MEXICO

We run on the "track" on the upper deck of the boat. We run loops. We run past the bar multiple times and past the smoking section multiple times. At one point, an inebriated guy calls out "Clear the way, clear the way—people taking care of themselves coming through!" Ha, ha. It feels that way—and it feels good.

We end our run at the gym with another mile on the treadmill. It's cooler than yesterday and the music is still sh*tty but at least it isn't as loud.

DAY 248. SATURDAY, JANUARY 9. COZUMEL, MEXICO

Feeling healthy in a sea (bad pun) of people who are indulging and some, overindulging.

TIP: Run no matter what the people around you are doing! Running will keep you grounded in the midst of it all.

Yay for running and good health! Now for the beach!

DAY 249. SUNDAY, JANUARY 10. ON THE HIGH SEAS— I CAN SEE CUBA FROM HERE.

Matt and I make a treadmill sandwich around monster musician Mike Dillon who is running between us. I love seeing musicians who spend so much time on the road staying healthy. There's a reason Mike is unafraid to tear his shirt off in the middle of a show. He takes care of himself, and apparently it's working for him—and for the rest of us too!

DAY 250. MONDAY, JANUARY 11. PORTLAND, OR

A late, late party night, off the boat and onto one plane and then another. My butt is so tired of sitting. It's spritzing snowy rain when we get back and almost midnight in island time and we need to get the run in. As soon as I head out, I'm wet and I miss the sand and sun. Matt says he feels heavy, and I have to go to the bathroom. Still, it's so good to get the fresh air and to move. Running while on the road really helped me stay grounded. Now that I'm back, it's helping me reintegrate. That and a good night sleep tonight plus a run in the morning and I'll be rocking it.

DAY 251. TUESDAY, JANUARY 12. PORTLAND, OR

Travel. It's hard to keep nutrition, digestion, sleep, rest, exercise, all of it, on an even keel when you are on the road and moving fast. Running is the consistency that is keeping it all in check for me. Getting out this morning is helping me adjust. Keeping it going is the ticket.

DAY 252. WEDNESDAY, JANUARY 13. PORTLAND, OR

Three miles in the pouring rain, and I don't know why but I can't peel the smile off my face. The run feels great even though I am so soaked by the time I get back that my underwear is completely stuck to my body! A happy run in the rain for the win!

DAY 253. THURSDAY, JANUARY 14. PORTLAND, OR

My Garmin says today was my fastest 5k...fastest 5k since starting tracking with my Garmin, which is to say fastest 5k over a vacation to Mexico, a couple of snow days, a cruise, and my vacation recovery days. In other words, probably not my fastest 5k *ever*, but I'll take it! Boom.

DAY 254. FRIDAY, JANUARY 15. PORTLAND, OR

I get the kids out the door early today and sit down to read the news online for a few minutes. You can probably tell where this is going! Those few minutes turn into a few more, and I almost miss the window to get out the door. I cut my run short by a mile because I'm compressed for time.

TIP: If you want to get out for a morning run, don't allow yourself any news or online time until AFTER the run. Ever.

DAY 255. SATURDAY, JANUARY 16. PORTLAND, OR

Wait long enough to go out on a Saturday morning and you'll see 10 times the number of runners that you see on a regular weekday morning run. I love the runner's wave or head nod as we pass each other.

I am seriously huffing at the end of this run and am certain it is my fastest yet. It isn't. Just the hardest. And this is the way it goes.

DAY 256. SUNDAY, JANUARY 17. PORTLAND, OR

I love my Sunday runs! Five miles in the pouring rain. If I take it slower I feel like I can go and go. Aaaaah.

DAY 257. MONDAY, JANUARY 18. PORTLAND, OR

I am trying to do at least three miles a day this year. I hit most of that three on the track today. Sometimes going 'round and 'round makes me crazy and sometimes, like today, it's just the thing to allow my body to relax and my thoughts be spacious.

DAY 258. TUESDAY, JANUARY 19. PORTLAND, OR

Dark o'clock. I love how the numbers of days of the streak just keep creeping up there. I guess that what you get with consistency! Matt said it smelled like snow out there this morning but I think snow and wet, sloppy rain kind of smell the same.

DAY 259. WEDNESDAY, JANUARY 20. PORTLAND, OR

When I take a slower pace I feel I can go and go. I am consistently knocking out at least three miles for a mini streak within the streak[5] now.

DAY 260. THURSDAY, JANUARY 21. PORTLAND, OR

TIP: And the running lesson for today is…always check the weather forecast before you go out. Trust me on this one. Then, check to make sure your tracking mechanism is charged too.

It got unexpectedly warm here overnight but I dressed for the colder days we've been having. I couldn't understand why my head was so sweaty under my baseball hat. Duh!

Of course, one good lesson deserves another. After my Garmin notifies me that I've hit my first mile with a buzz to my wrist, it keeps buzzing and begins to shut down. Why is it so disappointing to run miles that don't get logged?!

---

5   A streak within the streak is when you add an additional daily commitment like running a minimum of five miles a day instead of one, or adding a number of pushups to each day's workout.

> Do you have hatitude?
>
> I have a variety of **hats**—baseball hats, trucker hats, skullcaps, fuzzy hats, visors—that I rotate wearing depending on the weather, or sometimes I go without. Too much hat makes for a sweaty head, but some days call for wind protection, some days for sun protection and some days for nothing at all. It's a pretty personal choice.

DAY 261. FRIDAY, JANUARY 22. PORTLAND, OR

You know it's early when it's still dark after you return from your run! Nice pace today. Feeling fast and fit!

DAY 262. SATURDAY, JANUARY 23. PORTLAND, OR

I get out for my run early, followed by a romp with the dogs at the dog park. The minute we walk in the door it starts dumping rain. Like when the weather is crappy at home while you're on a tropical vacation, I take mild satisfaction in this!

I have an ache and tiny bump growing on my left big toe joint I've been ignoring. I suspect a bunion is forming. My runs often move me to action so when I come back today I book an appointment with Dr. Ray. It's not for another month, and I plan to take extra-exquisite care of my feet until then.

DAY 263. SUNDAY, JANUARY 24. PORTLAND, OR

I love the spaciousness of a Sunday run when I don't have to rush back for a kid activity. Matt joins me today. His pace is slower than mine, but he runs farther than he has run in years—yay! I love running with him *and* this introvert also cherishes the meditation and clarity that kicks in when I am solo. Good to balance the two! Another five mile Sunday in the books.

DAY 264. MONDAY, JANUARY 25. PORTLAND, OR

We're skiing today so I head out early to get my run in. As I am looping the track I contemplate breaking my streak within the streak (I've been consistent about running at least three miles daily and often more for most of this month instead of the one mile required by the US Streak Runners organization) because I want to save my legs for skiing.

Then I think about the mental edge I read about in *How Bad Do You Want it?* and that helps me set that reservation aside and maintain the mini streak, too.

DAY 265. TUESDAY, JANUARY 26. PORTLAND, OR

I love these early morning runs when it's misty outside. It feels so good on my face. I feel strong, and the minimum three miles go quickly. Not feeling fatigued from running and skiing yesterday either—only energized! Booyah!

DAY 266. WEDNESDAY, JANUARY 27. PORTLAND, OR

I find my mind wandering to thoughts of trail runs and ultras while I am out this morning. I run a 5k route and imagine doing that same loop four, nine, or nineteen more times to make the ultra-distance lengths of 25, 50, or 100k. In some ways I think I can imagine it, but it's probably like imagining what it's like to give birth before you do it. You can imagine all you want, but until you do it…Still, a girl can dream.

DAY 267. THURSDAY, JANUARY 28. SAN FRANCISCO, CA

I get to the hotel gym, and it's completely dark. I step in and find the light. It's a decent hotel but this gym leaves a lot to be desired. The treadmill looks like they ordered it from the back of a comic book. I get a couple of miles in, but I feel unsettled the whole time and decide to cut it short. It's really early and no one else is around. Something just doesn't feel right and I don't feel entirely safe.

As I am leaving, I have to pass the bank where they have computers to print your boarding pass which I can see from the gym door and…there's a guy at the desk looking at porn and jerking off. Seriously. I rattle the gym door so he knows he's not alone, and I beeline it to the elevator. Ugh. I don't get home until late tonight but I want to do this run over—and to preserve my 5k streak within the streak. What a way to start the day. It can only go up from here…right?

TIP: To all the runners—especially the women—be safe out there, wherever you are. Seriously, take precautions and trust your gut.

DAY 268. FRIDAY, JANUARY 29. PORTLAND, OR

I was not able to keep my 5k streak within a streak by running when I got home last night, so I restart it today. This morning's run in the rain is therapeutic as it gives me the spaciousness to really think about what happened yesterday and the lack of any real response or action on the part of the hotel. Ugh. And…onward!

DAY 269. SATURDAY, JANUARY 30. PORTLAND, OR

I can't always pinpoint why but some months my period just whoops my ass. Today is one of those days that feels like a massacre in my pants. I get in my 5k and feel like I am dragging around the whole time but…I'm still happy to be out, to be consistent, to get exercise and fresh air, and a clean perspective. Apparently, I need it!

PROGRESS REPORT: Holy moly! Less than 100 days now to hit my year mark!

DAY 270. SUNDAY, JANUARY 31. PORTLAND, OR

A lovely 5k to start my birthday and then heading to the slopes with the whole famdamily. My happy place!

DAY 271. MONDAY, FEBRUARY 1. PORTLAND, OR

Still feeling the warm fuzzies from my birthday yesterday. Weekend birthdays are the best! After running 5k followed by a day of skiing, I had that happy exhaustion thing going on last night. My legs feel fresh this morning, though, and I have a good, happy 5k to start the day in my new birthday socks!

DAY 272. TUESDAY, FEBRUARY 2. PORTLAND, OR

It rained yesterday and got cold enough overnight that there is an ever-so-thin sheet of ice covering the roads this morning—the kind that you don't really see, or if you do you don't think it will be that big of a deal, but it's deceivingly treacherous. So, today's run is a bit of a shuffle, especially at the higher elevation points. I do see the whole setup of tractor-trailers and tents, etc. for where they are shooting a TV series in the neighborhood. That's always interesting. And the security guards all wave as I shuffle by.

DAY 273. WEDNESDAY, FEBRUARY 3. PORTLAND, OR

An unexpected and important early morning call could have waylaid my running plans, but everyone in the family is so accustomed to my routine now that we just correct course and make it happen.

When I get to the track one of the runners says to me, "You're late!" I reply, "I know, so I'd better run fast!" This guy, he's a regular, and I know now that his name is Greg. He is out there rain or shine. The first time I ever saw him I was walking my daughter to school through the park. He'd just left the track. His shorts were so torn up you could see his underwear in several spots. He just looked crazy and...I remember clearly, I steered my daughter away from walking behind him.

Fast-forward a couple of years and I am seeing this guy on the track every day. He's steady and determined. One day

I see him at yoga class. He's the only guy without a mat, and his toenails look like they haven't been cut in years. For all intents and purposes he looks like a guy that has just rolled off of the street, and maybe he has, but, man, he works out hard! And consistently. And he's the friendliest face on the track every morning. We acknowledge each other every time. He remembers my name, and Matt's. I love this friendly banter. And I love that someone I once steered far away from was my biggest cheerleader this morning.

Running unites.

DAY 274. THURSDAY, FEBRUARY 4. PORTLAND, OR

Argh! I lost today's run info on my Garmin this morning. I'm not sure how I did it or how relatable this would be for non-runners, but I find this blank spot in my calendar of consistency so frustrating. Other than this first world issue though—thank God I got to run today!

DAY 275. FRIDAY, FEBRUARY 5. PORTLAND

It snowed hard on the mountain yesterday—it really was a blizzard. With **so much** deep, wet powder on the mountain I was WAY out of my league. All of the things I usually do that make me feel like a badass out on the slopes weren't working in that kind of snow. It was deep and heavy and I couldn't control my speed or turns and…as a result, I fell. A lot. I morphed from that badass into a big, snotty, tired, frustrated, banged-up, baby sitting chest deep in the snow on the mountain.

As a result of yesterday's misadventures I feel like I have whiplash. My neck is a wreck and my shoulders and upper back aren't much better. Somehow though, being straight and upright and moving forward is working ok, so I get in my 5k plus some this morning. Matt quits after the first lap at the track because his knee is bothering him. Today, we feel like two old people complaining about our ailments. I am grateful that most days don't feel like this.

DAY 276. SATURDAY, FEBRUARY 6. PORTLAND

Got some bodywork yesterday. My neck is just totally seized up. Side to side is okay but up and down—forget about it! Matt cautions me to take it easy this morning, maybe just get a mile in. I wear a neck warmer—my body worker said that heat is really important; to let it sweat during the run and not to let it get cold.

During the first half-mile or so, I can really feel the stiffness and think I might cut it short but something about moving helps loosen things up too. My whole body feels like it has been beat up, but I get in a nice and easy three miles before calling it quits. Today's pace is perhaps more like a jog than a run, but it's a good lesson in just getting out there. Onward towards the healing—and beware the deep, heavy powder!

DAY 277. SUNDAY, FEBRUARY 7. PORTLAND

Amazingly my neck started to really loosen up yesterday afternoon. I've had my neck warmer on 24 hours/day minus the Epsom salt baths.

I decided to get back on the skis because I had the opportunity to do so with the whole family. And I decided not to run first so my legs would be fresher for skiing, which seemed to work in my favor. We had an epic day of skiing.

We return home, unpack, and I put on my running stuff and head out. I can surely say that in the past I would have thought skiing was enough exercise for one day and that would have been that but...we know how that goes these days! A 20-year high for warm temperatures surprised me today and I was way over overdressed—especially with my cozy neck warmer. Amazingly, my legs feel relatively fresh and even though the run feels like a bit of a slog I am pleased to see on my Garmin that my pace is right in there with my usual morning run pace. Winning!

DAY 278. MONDAY, FEBRUARY 8. PORTLAND, OR

Today I break in a new pair of happy socks I got for my birthday. You just can't help but smile when you wear these ridiculous things—great for enhancing and elevating a mood.

I am spending more and more time online looking at and learning about ultras and thinking about mixing up my daily 5k with some longer and shorter runs to start training for longer distances. Did I just say that?! Yikes!

DAY 279. TUESDAY, FEBRUARY 9. PORTLAND, OR

We are entering into a family zone of nonstop travel for the next few weeks so I am feeling extra gratitude and appreciation for the consistency of the running streak as everything else swirls around. Another 5k to start the day in the books.

DAY 280. WEDNESDAY, FEBRUARY 10. DENVER, CO

I got up at 3:00 a.m. Portland time to get my miles in before starting my meeting day here. By 5:30 a.m. Denver time the gym is full—and full of men. I count 16 from the time I arrive until I leave and only one other woman who arrives as I leave. It's always encouraging when a hotel gym is packed first thing in the morning, but I'm left wondering where my ladies are. Regardless, my 5k on the treadmill sets a great tone for a full day.

DAY 281. THURSDAY, FEBRUARY 11. PORTLAND, OR

Good to be back home. It's starting to feel like spring out there, and I really appreciated being outside again after yesterday's treadmill run. I experiment with running in a new running skirt and am not yet convinced it's the way to go. I hate how running tights leave so little to the imagination but don't really care for the restriction of the skirt either.

I met a guy yesterday who is an ultra-marathoner. He lives near trails not far from where I once lived in West Marin, California, and spends lots of time on those trails—more as a meditation than anything else. I am witnessing myself feeling envious of and longing for that!

SHORTS, TIGHTS, SKORTS, SKIRTS

The model of **Sporthill Shorts** I have is so old I don't think they make them any longer, but they've lasted forever and they're still my all time favorite shorts.

My favorite thing to wear on my lower half are **capri length running tights**. I now have some from **Nike, Prana**, and **Sportskirts** and some cheaper brands I found on a discount rack at Marshalls. I like them all although I feel like tights leave little to the imagination, particularly in the posterior. For really cold days, I have some longer tights.

To help cover my ass, literally, I also wear running **skirts and skorts** and after some experimentation have some new favorites from **Mountain Hardwear, Lululemon**, and **Prana** with my most favorites coming from **Sportskirts**.

There are so many decisions to make: color, style, length, with brief or shorts or tights built in, with nothing built in, and so on. If I had 100 pairs I'd wear them all, but ultimately while all this stuff is awesome when it's fresh and clean, it doesn't stay that way for long. It all gets sweaty and dirty and really is there just to support you to get the job done—so my advice is to use whatever works!

DAY 282. FRIDAY, FEBRUARY 12. PORTLAND, OR

It is just shy of 50 degrees this morning when I head out. Hope the snow on the mountain isn't melting just yet. These running legs want to ski some more too!

Today I run around the park in the grass and on the dirt trails to simulate trail running. I notice that when I run on the street and especially the track that I can let my mind wander but the dirt really forces me to pay attention to where I place my feet—different kind of awareness.

Running on different surfaces is an awareness practice.

DAY 283. SATURDAY, FEBRUARY 13. BRIGHTWOOD, OR

I'm running country roads with lots of hills and beautiful scenery early this morning. I'm trying compression socks for the first time and loving the way they make my calves feel. In fact, I wish I could have a full body compression suit! On my run I discover a park with dirt trails and come back to it later in the day for a hike with the kids.

DAY 284. SUNDAY, FEBRUARY 14. BRIGHTWOOD, OR

It poured all night long, and it's just dumping this morning. I imagine the lovely trails I discovered yesterday are now little muddy rivers, so instead I take to the road again. I think I've picked up about five pounds of water weight in my soggy shoes and clothes. Still, the scenery is beautiful and the hills are the right kind of challenge.

81 days until the one-year mark. I look back in my log to see where I was at on Day 81. Matt was resting his knee, I

was doing some hills, and it was a spacious Sunday run. Déjà vu all over again—in the very best of ways!

DAY 285. MONDAY, FEBRUARY 15. PORTLAND, OR

Back home and out the door first thing for 5k before heading to the airport. I always love my pre-flight runs and imagine I'll be hankering for one post-flight too.

Although it's mid-February, my run this morning is filled with blooming camellias, daffodils, crocuses (I just had to say crocuses because the real plural of the word—croci—sounds not like a cute little flower) and blooming trees. Witnessing this is just one of the many bonuses of traveling by foot!

DAY 286. TUESDAY, FEBRUARY 16. CHICAGO, IL

During my run this morning I can't stop thinking about all of the runners in the LA Marathon and in the US Olympic Marathon trials that took place over the weekend. At the trials and during the marathon, the temperature soared—higher than it had ever been for the trials. As a result, many runners ended up overheating and/or dropping out due to the challenging conditions.

I'm running in a hotel gym in Chicago early this morning. It's snowing outside and the gym is 70 plus degrees. That's about 30 degrees warmer than my typical morning run and, as a result, I am feeling the warmth—in fact, my face looks like a big, giant beet by the time I'm done! Another one in the books.

DAY 287. WEDNESDAY, FEBRUARY 17. PORTLAND, OR

I'm feeling a little ragged this morning after my travels. There's a lack of rhythm in my run, and it is effortful. Still, it's good to be back at the track with the rest of the regulars.

DAY 288. THURSDAY, FEBRUARY 18. PORTLAND, OR

I'm solo parenting for the rest of the week and an early start day for the kids means getting up and out the door extra early. As it isn't as early as I might have liked, I run extra fast. I'm trying to look at my Garmin stats and frustrated that I don't know my way around my watch, phone, and online tracking better. I'm sure I'm missing something, but right now it's not feeling very intuitive. Ugh. #firstworldproblems

DAY 289. FRIDAY, FEBRUARY 19. PORTLAND, OR

I love the anecdote of the frog in the boiling pot of water. The premise is that if a frog is placed in a pot of boiling water it will jump out, but if it is placed in a pot of water that is cold and slowly heated then it won't notice what is coming and gets cooked to death.

I feel like the frog in the pot—but in a good way. I first got into this challenge with the minimum commitment of one mile. A significant factor in that commitment was that not only was it a manageable distance for me, it also wouldn't take much time. It wouldn't be a huge struggle to make that space in my day. Now, as time has gone by and my daily distance on a minimum day has tripled, so has the time commitment. Still, I seem to be managing fitting it in—whereas the thought of committing to a minimum of 30 minutes of running daily at the start would have been fairly overwhelming. Very sneaky.

> My new **CEP** compression socks rock. How can these funny little sleeves instantly make your legs feel happy? I don't know how it works, but it does and I'm loving it.

DAY 290. SATURDAY, FEBRUARY 20. PORTLAND, OR

I didn't eat very well yesterday or get as much sleep as I might have liked. Perhaps that's why after the first mile I sense my pace slowing down. I leave the track before I do my desired miles to run the neighborhood in a route that is unpredictable just to keep my mind engaged and body moving forward. Lots of early spring flowers to enjoy help keep me engaged too!

DAY 291. SUNDAY, FEBRUARY 21. PORTLAND, OR

There are very few things I miss about living in Eugene, Oregon, but the barkchip running trails is a big one. Today I head to the park in Portland with the closest approximation—a part dirt, part big, lumpy woodchip trail. I am happy to run around the park but I really despise the old cement street I have to take to reach it—the surface is just so hard on the body. I probably run a good gingerly mile on it, and that is a mile more than I would like. Guess you've got to take the good with the bad!

DAY 292. MONDAY, FEBRUARY 22. PORTLAND, OR

PROGRESS REPORT: Holy moly—getting close to 300 days! How is that possible?!

My 5k to start the day feels fast and good. I think after yesterday's hills and varied terrain that today's flat run to the park and track and around the neighborhood feels easy so I push it hard. I'm looking forward to running on some trails this coming weekend in Austin.

This past weekend I watched a few short videos about inspiring ultra-runners and races and may have even bookmarked a website for Ultra signups. Shhh....

Warning: Hanging out on UltraSignup is highly addictive as you learn about all the adventure that awaits you as a runner!

DAY 293. TUESDAY, FEBRUARY 23. PORTLAND, OR

Wow—what an amazing, giant moon! Noticing that and the sound of multiple people scraping their windshields of ice during my early morning run. The daffodils are blooming, but the frost is back. It's a packed day today. I'm so glad I'm getting to run this morning!

DAY 294. WEDNESDAY, FEBRUARY 24. PORTLAND, OR

I'm rising and getting out the door earlier and earlier this week with a dark o'clock run down my usual Sunday route this morning. There's no traffic this early and with a busy week ahead this was another perfect start to help balance the day. Boom!

DAY 295. THURSDAY, FEBRUARY 25. PORTLAND, OR

Running in the correct shoe is key.
—Bill Rodgers, Four-time Boston Marathon Winner

I went to see star podiatrist, Dr. Ray, today after my run. He is the bomb! I'm so glad I went and had my neuromas checked—he even had his medical student come over and check them out because it's unusual to have a double right where mine are (lucky me!). He did a bunion massage that kicked my arse—or foot, as it may be—and some debridement on one of my toenails. Runners often have gross toenails. What can I say?

I learn so much from him and a big one today was realizing that I actually am running on bone, which is why my feet feel so sensitive. It's not because I'm getting older; rather, it's a readjustment of the fat pad under the ball of my feet due to the stress and tightness of the nerve tissue around the neuromas and bunion pathway. I've got stretches to do, self-massage to administer, and am back in my Correct Toe spacers to help with that now.

One service that Dr. Ray offers that I love is to bring your footwear to him to check out. He'll help make adjustments (often cutting into a pair to make them roomier) or give recommendations on how to do it yourself. Unless you're a barefoot runner, there's no piece of gear more critical to a runner than their footwear. It pays to get it right.

TIP: Happy feet make for a happy runner.

Warning: Happy runners love to buy running shoes. Lots and lots of running shoes.

MY YEAR IN SHOES

I started the streak with **Nike** *Free*, and I'm still a fan. I know the trail community scoffs at people who run in Nikes—it often seems like a brand of activewear that people wear when they're not being particularly active. However…Nike *Frees* have a toe box that's wider than many models of shoes that claim to be wide toe box, and that's a really important feature to me. I have a couple of pairs that I rotate.

I bought my first pair of **Altras** (the *Intuition* model), brought them to Dr. Ray, along with my *Frees*, and we pulled the insole out of each to compare side by side. My foot was nicely inside the outline of the Nike Free insole with plenty of wiggle room while my toes were hanging over the Altra insole, meaning my feet were going to get squished inside those shoes, which, mile after mile, is a really big deal. Disappointing from a company known for its wide toe box.

However, I've become a *huge* fan of my **Altra** *Ones*. Some people think they look like clown shoes (and they're right!), but I love the roominess in the toes. I really didn't notice the adjustment to the zero drop (shoes that have a level profile on the bottom and no "drop" from the heel to the front of the shoe), perhaps because my Nikes were so flat already.

I wear my running shoes with **metatarsal pads** inside them to provide extra encouragement for my toes to spread out and ease away from my neuromas.

I've also invested in **Altra** *Superior* for my trail runs. I get the occasional black toenails when I trail race in them, but I've logged some awesomely satisfying trail miles.

DAY 296. FRIDAY, FEBRUARY 26. PORTLAND, OR

I have an early morning flight, so I am out the door to run in the wee hours—and somehow it just doesn't feel like a big deal. I was so looking forward to running in my new shoes and they do not disappoint.

Four more days until 300! 10 times as many days as I set out to do originally.

DAY 297. SATURDAY, FEBRUARY 27. AUSTIN, TX

It's another one of those mornings when I look at my Garmin and it hasn't yet changed time zones and therefore reminds me that I am running at 3:00 or 4:00 a.m. in my home time zone. It's cold, it's dark, but…I've got wide-open trails to run here in Austin, and I am stoked. 5k on the trail for the win before a big board meeting day.

DAY 298. SUNDAY, FEBRUARY 28. AUSTIN, TX

It's warmer this morning. I have mixed emotions—I got my 5k in and don't want to say goodbye to the trails and head back to the pavement, but I feel kind of achy and ragged and am ready to go home.

DAY 299. MONDAY, FEBRUARY 29. PORTLAND, OR

I came home with the flu last night. I cancelled my meetings and stayed in bed most of the day. I'm generally so healthy, or maybe it's stubborn, that I literally cannot remember if I have ever done that before. I felt really awful all day—just the worst—headache, cough, sore throat, fever of about 1,000 degrees, sinus pain…you name it.

It is really hard to stand up, let alone get out the door but there is no question that I just have to do it. And wouldn't you know, just like when you feel fine, getting out helps you feel even better—even when the going is sloooow. I keep the streak alive with my slowest mile ever but break the streak within the streak of at least 5k. That was definitely not going to happen.

TIP: Streaking while sick? Sometimes running can make you feel better when you don't feel well. Be cautious and listen to your body.

DAY 300. TUESDAY, MARCH 1. PORTLAND, OR

The last two days have been the hardest yet to get out the door—achy, fevery, etc. Once I am out my legs feel like they're ready to go and go, but my lungs and the rest of my body isn't having it. Another super slow one—and it did help me feel better, though better is a relative term! Keeping the streak alive.

DAY 301. WEDNESDAY, MARCH 2. PORTLAND, OR

I am instantly winded as I run down the street. Even though I'm weak, my muscles feel fit but my lungs and heaving belly tell another story. Still, the air feels good on my face and I'm so grateful I can move.

DAY 302. THURSDAY, MARCH 3. PORTLAND, OR

I actually make it down to the park for a lap around the track but not much more. I have lost some weight being sick and my appetite has not fully returned. It must be some combination of my weight, my new lighter shoes, the lack of any real running the last few days, but I somehow feel light and fast and fit even while my respiratory system struggles. Or maybe it's just not feeling like total hell. My mile comes in around the nine-minute mark—certainly shorter and slower than usual but it encourages me. Just can't wait to get fully back in this game! So grateful it's waiting for me on the other side. Truth.

DAY 303. FRIDAY, MARCH 4. PORTLAND, OR

I think I'll feel like I'm back when I can get out for a morning run. I've just been feeling full of crud this week in the mornings and not ready for even a mile until later in the day. Tonight's run has me full of side stitches (typical for me when there's food in my system) and coughing, but just happy to be back out here. Aiming for more of this tomorrow and first thing.

DAY 304. SATURDAY, MARCH 5. PORTLAND, OR

I slept in much longer than I imagined the dogs would let me. Rising after them is how I can tell I'm not fully back yet among the land of the living. Last night I had a coughing fit so intense I thought I was going to cough up a lung. That is actually what it felt like—and my stomach too.

I get a couple of miles in at the park; the longest run all week. I have a race coming up in a week and am planning on firing on all cylinders by then. Right? Right?!

DAY 305. SUNDAY, MARCH 6. PORTLAND, OR

It's an early start for Calliope's soccer game, and I am all out of sorts without my morning run. It's gotten to be such a habit that it feels strange when it's not happening. I'm solo parenting and still not feeling 100%. I don't get out the door to run until after the day's activities and helping kids with homework and carpool. It's cold out, and I decide I don't really like running at night. A woman on a bike comes up from behind and scares the bejeezus out of me. Oh well. Another one in the books.

TIP: Bikers: Be kind to the runners on the road, and let them know you are coming up behind them before you are right on top of them lest they jump out of their skin! I may or may not know someone who has had this experience.

DAY 306. MONDAY, MARCH 7. PORTLAND, OR

I get out first thing this morning and feel like I'm starting all over again. The muscle memory is there, but my cardiovascular is compromised and since my appetite isn't back all the way yet I just feel kind of weak—like a 90-pound weakling. One day at a time.

DAY 307. TUESDAY, MARCH 8. PORTLAND, OR

Today marks the first time in over a week I've gotten the full 5k in. My legs, particularly my quads, feel fatigued. Does wearing compression socks on your lower legs fatigue your upper legs, or am I just pooped from coughing my lungs out all day long?

DAY 308. WEDNESDAY, MARCH 9. PORTLAND, OR

Yes! I managed another few miles today but overall I'm whupped. I'm working full speed ahead but still feeling like I'm not firing on all cylinders. I am ready for the sun to come out and to feel more robust. I'll take these miles though!

DAY 309. THURSDAY, MARCH 10. PORTLAND, OR

Three miles three days in a row. My chest still feels heavy and is full of junk. There's lots of coughing and I'm completely drained by the end of the day, but it is improving every day, to be sure. Grateful.

DAY 310. FRIDAY, MARCH 11. PORTLAND, OR

Even a toad has four ounces of strength.
—Chinese proverb

Still feeling wiped out. I went to sleep again at 9:00 p.m. last night. Matt cautions me not to run too far or fast and I don't—a relatively easy mile and a half. I feel fine when I'm outside and running, but I'm not fine the rest of the day. I need to rest up and kick this thing!

DAY 311. SATURDAY, MARCH 12. PORTLAND, OR

Just another short and easy one to the park and around the upper track today. The weather is really crappy—cold, damp, rainy, and I am just not firing on all cylinders. I am ready to be done with this thing that seems to have a hold on me. Tomorrow, I run five miles for the Shamrock Run 8k. I haven't run five miles straight since January 24. So much for training for this run!

DAY 312. SUNDAY, MARCH 13. SHAMROCK RUN. DOWNTOWN PORTLAND, OR

It is pouring, pouring, pouring, and cold and crappy. Really couldn't be much worse. The difference here between and 5k and 8k is that the runners are much more serious—few walkers or super slow pokes. My pace is good right from the start and I feel energetic and strong the whole way through. It may actually help that I'm already drenched and so cold at the start that I can't feel my feet because my body temperature adjusts quickly and I become just warm enough. Even though I've been low energy and feeling kind of crappo for weeks now and even though it's pouring icy rain and even though I haven't run 5 miles or more since January, or perhaps because of it all, I have a great 8k run.

That was the good stuff. The not so great was that Matt felt so crappy in the knee that he decided in the jog over to the start line that he was going to pass on the 5k in its entirety. The kids ran the 5k. Neither had a really great race, but they were good. It was cold, pouring and the course was full of puddles. I could have wrung out every article of clothing I was wearing and filled a bucket. But…in all the times we've run races we have been fortunate to miss the heavy rain. Multiple times it's poured all night, let up just before the run for the race and then begun pouring again after. We've seen lots of rainbows and sunshine. So…all in all, lots to be thankful for.

AND…yesterday we went to the US Indoor Track and Field Championships. Wow, wow, wow. So in awe of the athleticism and dedication of these tremendous athletes. What a production, too! If you ever get the chance….go! And if you get the chance to volunteer, like we did, even better!

DAY 313. MONDAY, MARCH 14. PORTLAND, OR

I read something last week that I thought was funny—something like a recovery run is still a run—just a run the day after a race. Really, a 5-mile run doesn't call for a "recovery" run the next day, but I do take it easy this morning since I was drenched head to toe in freezing rain for hours yesterday, and I just want to be mindful of being gentle with my health.

Today is the first day after we set the clocks forward, and though I am out at my regular time not only is it pitch dark, there wasn't a single other person on the track. I can remember this week last year, too. It seems like it takes everyone about a week or so to adjust and get their rear ends out the door into the darkness again. I heard that California is considering abolishing daylight savings time. Can't say that I would miss it!

DAY 314. TUESDAY, MARCH 15. PORTLAND, OR

It is so dark when I get out the door this morning. I run uphill and around the neighborhood. My feet can feel that I've been wearing my Correct Toes for a bit every day. The bunion zone is on alert—but I can tell that the toe spacers are doing their work. Grateful for that.

I volunteered with Calliope last night at the rehearsal for the World Indoor Track Championship opening ceremony. It was exciting to be behind the scenes—to see where the athletes would warm up and congregate and to just witness the tremendous production that happens behind the scenes. In my producer mode I couldn't help but see things that I would improve *but* I was in awe of what they were accomplishing together.

There is more track on the agenda this week: a parent meeting for Shea's track team, Shea's first track meet of the season, the opening ceremonies for the World Indoor Championships and Shea's participation as a volunteer in the meet all weekend.

DAY 315. WEDNESDAY, MARCH 16. PORTLAND, OR

Daylight savings time is kicking my butt. At night, I'm wide-awake when I should be going to bed, and then I am dragging my ass out of bed in the morning. It was a late start for my run this morning, and my Garmin beeped afterwards to inform me that one of the miles was my fastest yet (since I've been using my Garmin, of course). It wasn't until later that I realized I had drunk my tea before heading out the door this morning, which is something I very rarely do. I have a sneaking suspicion that the morning caffeine acted like a performance-enhancing drug. Still, I suppose I should be happy about the whole deal. It's not like anyone's going to test me!

> I bought a **foam roller** today. It's not torture if it's in the name of physical therapy, right?!
>
> Apparently this is now how I roll! Yuk, yuk...

DAY 316. SAINT PATRICK'S DAY, THURSDAY, MARCH 17. PORTLAND, OR

Brrrr...so cold this morning. The sun came out yesterday for the first time in what felt like forever, but when it's clear it's cold and there is frost on the rooftops this morning. Daylight savings time still has me dragging in the morning, and I am still feeling the remnants of my illness so I get out the door late, which means more people and traffic and just a choppier run.

I see Greg, my running pal, on the track. He's one of those people who just has a great attitude. When I mention the cold, he holds his arms up to the sky like he is giving thanks and says, "You're out here!" Enough said.

DAY 317. FRIDAY, MARCH 18. PORTLAND, OR

Windy, windy, windy. Since I signed up for a trail run in early April that has 1500 feet in elevation gain and because I primarily run on the flats, I want to get some hills in today.

This takes me to an area not far from my neighborhood that I rarely get to but just love—beautiful homes, lovely gardens, little hidden lanes. Right around the halfway point my digestive system starts telling me I shouldn't have had that giant froyo at the World Indoor Track meet last night. One advantage of running in the woods is pooping in the forest if the need arises. No bushes to duck behind around here. All in all a decent run—especially once I'd make it home!

DAY 318. SATURDAY, MARCH 19. PORTLAND, OR

There was a post recently in one of my online running groups about what kind of underwear women might or might not be wearing while they run. The consensus of that group, at least as they were telling it online, was that most of them run commando. Whatever your choice, in my mind however, there is for most of us women about one week out of every month when that preference really doesn't work.

Speaking of online groups…it used to be that I would jump onto social media and catch up with what was going on with my family and extended circle of friends. These days, I belong to so many running groups that my feeds are fully populated with all things running—trails and roads, races and shoes, running nutrition and hydration, inspiration and support…and while I don't actually know a single one of these people, they're my online community. It's kind of strange but definitely sweet—with lots of spunk thrown in there too!

Shea volunteered yesterday and today at the World Indoor Track Meet. I met a guy while I was there the other day who travelled from Germany so that he could volunteer. What an amazing and inspiring experience—right in our own backyard.

A WORD ABOUT RUNNING WHILE MENSTRUATING

After numerous runs in which my panties and my period protection were all in a bunch I've become a fan of **THINX** period protection sport undies. I've been digging some of their other styles for day and nighttime wear, eliminating or reducing the need for tampons and pads, etc. but find them a little bulky under my running tights. The sport version is better but it's still not a perfect option. I don't know of one yet.

Most female trail runners I know struggle with this issue. If you use tampons or pads and you pack in and out, in addition to your clean supplies you end up running with bloody "hygiene" products in your hydration vest too. Not to mention the time lost while you are managing this stuff.

For years I'd been hearing about women who swear by the **Diva Cup**—a sort of cervical cap which collects your monthly fluid and can keep you going hours longer than tampons or pads before being washed and reinserted. I'm a new convert and love the additional freedom but on heavier days and longer runs it can be challenging to contend with out on the trail or road or in any bathroom that's not the comfort of your own home.

This is clearly one place where innovation is needed! We have thousands of options for running shoes and other gear but only a few options for an issue that is part of most women's lives for years and years, and an issue especially challenging for athletes. OK, it's challenging for all of us who bleed, which is most of us. I wish I had better solutions.

DAY 319. SUNDAY, MARCH 20. PORTLAND, OR

Never wipe your ass with a squirrel.
—Jason Robillard

Well, crap! It's the second time this week my run is being interrupted by, well…crap. I get to about my halfway point in the run and nature is *calling*. Again, I'm not on a trail but in a neighborhood and I have fantasies of starting an app where runners could open their bathrooms to each other if the need strikes during a run. I walk home, take care of business, and head out to complete my mileage. Not my favorite run, but another one in the books.

DAY 320. MONDAY, MARCH 21. PORTLAND, OR

It's the first weekday of spring break, and I'm loving how I can get out the door a little later but not have the usual school traffic to contend with. There are several spring break boot camp groups working out at the park who make me realize that what I do isn't difficult at all. I'm not sure they're enjoying themselves as much as I am, but I wouldn't mind being more fit in the upper body and flexible too.

DAY 321. TUESDAY, MARCH 22. GOVERNMENT CAMP, OR

It snowed last night, it's snowing right now, and the temperature is much lower than it is for my usual run. Even though it's cold, I am warm—too warm. The combination of uphill right out the door, too much wine last night and being way overdressed makes me feel uncomfortable and overheated. And…it's beautiful outside, we're on spring break, the snow is soft and squeaky underfoot, and I am so fortunate. Next, to ski!

DAY 322. WEDNESDAY, MARCH 23. GOVERNMENT CAMP, OR

I woke up this morning and read some ultra-running blogs relating experiences of running 100-mile races. So inspiring—both the runners and their support teams. It's good stuff to fill my head with.

It's a little warmer than yesterday. The ground is both snowy and slushy and my shoes are definitely not made for running in this stuff, but I don't care. I'm up and out early and not overdressed. There aren't too many—okay, any— runners around here. I'm thinking everyone saves all they have for the slopes.

I have an epic afternoon of skiing after my morning meetings and then an amazing early evening snowhike. Love, love, love these outdoor active days! Yes!

DAY 323. THURSDAY, MARCH 24. GOVERNMENT CAMP, OR

Phew. With running, skiing and snowhiking yesterday, I feel like toast this morning. I'm bone tired, maybe a little hungover and not really feeling like running in the cold and windy air. *Of course*, I do it anyway—a quick but decent run on a layer of fresh, wet snow before heading up the mountain to hit it once again.

Also, I feel like I could eat a house right now. Related?

TIP: Running a lot means eating everything in site—guilt free! Winning!

DAY 324. FRIDAY, MARCH 25. GOVERNMENT CAMP, OR

Wow, wow, wow is it beautiful during my run! It snowed last night and it is still coming down this morning. We jump on the trail right near the cabin. The first half-mile is uphill and there is so much snow on the ground that it is *all* really challenging. A great workout in a spectacular location and my first run of the streak in my snow boots!

DAY 325. SATURDAY, MARCH 26. PORTLAND, OR

Spring has definitely sprung in Portland. It's amazing how much can happen in the natural world in just a few days. After running in the snow all week, my Altras feel like they are flying on the road and track, and it feels *good*!

DAY 326. EASTER SUNDAY, MARCH 27. PORTLAND, OR

> *My nose is running faster than I am!*
> —Me, this morning

Have you ever seen a cartoon of someone who has a faucet for a nose? That is me this morning. With everything blooming and all the pollen in the air I am a runny, running faucet. Ultra-runners always seem to talk about blowing snot rockets (lovely, I know, but it gets real out on the trail). However, a runny nose does not make for snot rocket material, only an annoyance. Still, grateful I have legs and feet to run, a nose to breathe, and a sleeve to wipe it on.

DAY 327. MONDAY, MARCH 28. PORTLAND, OR

I have a trail race to look forward to this weekend! There's nothing like a race to put a stake in the ground. I want to get some new trail shoes, but otherwise I think I'm covered. This morning on my run I am thinking about how appealing longer and longer distances are AND I'm thinking about how good it feels to be consistent and to have stayed injury free all year long. I have concerns about adding distance and mixing up my terrain. I'm just so happy to be able to do this much, but I do wonder…how much more could I do and still be in this sweet spot? That is the question.

Warning: The running streak has a way of sneaking up on you and pushing you towards bigger, better, higher, different aspirations.

DAY 328. TUESDAY, MARCH 29. PORTLAND, OR

I ordered my trail shoes from Zappos last night. I really like to support my local running stores, but this week a girl has got to do what a girl has got to do and Zappos does it fast! I'm getting excited to get out there on the trail. I also had a reminder that registration for a 50k trail run I just might be interested in is opening this week.

On my run I think back to my marathon training days, remembering the time commitment for the long runs, etc. and the obsession on my mind for the weeks leading up to them. I'm happy with my current level of fitness and that I've been able to run every single day for almost a year without injury.

Am I ready to risk that to grow?

DAY 329. WEDNESDAY, MARCH 30. PORTLAND, OR

One benefit of recovering from the daylight saving time switch is getting out early enough to see the sunrise. Spring has really sprung here, and it's our warmest week yet. The sun is a ball of fire in the sky this morning—so lovely. So many spring flowers too. I'm feeling strong and wishing I'd made time to start my day with more than just 5k, though I got in some hills in anticipation of this weekend's trail run. Loving my running!

DAY 330. THURSDAY, MARCH 31. PORTLAND, OR

I'm dragging my sorry ass during my run this morning. My arms feel heavy, my legs feel heavy, and I am tired.

When I push the button on my Garmin at the end I see that I've logged my second fastest time for a 5k all year. How is it possible I was really feeling like a slug and didn't realize I was running at that pace? I am scratching my head over this one.

Registration opens tomorrow for the Portland Trail Series, which feels like it would be a great challenge. It's got a limited field of runners that I suspect are way more experienced than I and great trails I want to get to know better, right here in Portland. Am I ready to commit to this?

TIP: As I'm running I'm thinking that some days you're just not feeling it and that's all part of it too. Just keep moving.

DAY 331. FRIDAY, APRIL 1. PORTLAND, OR

I guess I answered yesterday's question when I woke up this morning and jumped on registration for the Portland Trail Series just minutes after it opened. This series races five times over five weeks in the summer evenings on Portland's Forest Park trails.

The runs are five to seven miles long. Matt surprised me by saying he wanted to commit to it, too, so I got us both registered. I'm super excited to have a flag in the ground to get me onto those trails and to mix it up with this community too.

Last night I checked the map for my first trail race this weekend and, of course, finishing times from the last couple of years. When you look at the running times for trail runs when your head has been in road races it looks like everyone is moving at a snail's pace. When you look at the map of trails and the elevation gain (gulp!) you realize they're totally cooking out there.

For my run this morning I put hill repeats in—something I never do. It is fun charging down the shortcut to the bottom and heading up again and again…to a certain point. Then I start feeling a little apprehensive about this weekend's race. I know lots of runners, maybe even most, get nervous before races. To me, feeling this way means that I care. This is a good thing. Right?!

DAY 332. SATURDAY, APRIL 2. PORTLAND, OR

Today is the first run in my new trail shoes *and* in some new running tights. I love new gear! The weather is beautiful, and I am getting so excited about tomorrow's trail run and trail running in general.

Nature, trails…these are things deeply baked inside me. Matt and I hiked on our first date. I hiked on the days I gave birth to both of my children. In Eugene, we lived right off the barkchip trails where I trained for my first (and only) marathon 10 years ago. But since moving to Portland and enjoying a more urban lifestyle I have lost my connection to the trails. Trail running feels like it will bring that back, which makes me feel like I'm coming home to myself. Exhale.

A NOTE ABOUT RUNNING BRAS

It's hard to believe how expensive decent **running bras** are! Like the way that the majority of states tax tampons as a luxury item, it seems out of whack that such a wee bit of technical fabric could cost so darned much—and still be so hard to fit properly! Still, they're a necessary evil.

I've invested in a few from **Lululemon** and others in the $60 range but my favorite is a **Champion** bra I found on sale for $12 in Florida—I realized I was about to board a cruise ship for a week without a running bra in my possession and had my Uber driver pull over at a sporting goods store so I could pick one up. Since that time I've picked up a handful more and find them the most comfortable for me.

DAY 333. SUNDAY, APRIL 3. STUBB STEWART TRAIL CHALLENGE. BUXTON, OR

My first trail race today, and I am completely hooked!

Beautiful day, beautiful setting, nice people—no traffic or crowds. The course is challenging. The first mile is pretty much a straight shot up. It's hard but the reward on the other side is awesome—a long, loping trail with curves and ups and downs. I am flying through the forest and thinking about how much I want to just run in the forest for fun, not just to race.

In the parts where I'm not being seriously challenged my mind goes to so many places—really good, clear, creative thinking. Then comes the long, slow upward slope. Matt meets me along the way and runs for a bit. I can't talk with him at all I am heaving so hard. I wave him off and then the final mile is a killer straight up, like a kick when you are down. Argh! But…I do it all. I feel strong and happy. It is sunny. The views are epic. The dogs love being out in the park. We love being out here too. It's like giving birth; you kind of forget about how much it hurts afterwards! Well, this was actually nothing like childbirth but what I mean is that there is real reward that comes from pushing yourself, and I really had fun. More.of.this!

DAY 334. MONDAY, APRIL 4. PORTLAND, OR

I was glued to the Twitter feed for the Barkley Marathon[6] all weekend. I can't believe the final three runners are still out there. Two nights in a row I have gone to sleep while they were out there! I'm in serious awe of anyone who can go that far into beast mode. And I was feeling like a badass after completing a 10k trail run!

I haven't done a lot of racing so far this year, just a lot of steady running. In fact, I've already signed up for more races in the next few months than I ran all last year.

What is notable is that four of the road races I ran this year I had previously run for several years in a row, and my time for each one of them this year was a healthy PR (Personal record, my best time for a distance or race.).

---

6   Barkley Marathon—The race that eats its young. Check out the video on Netflix.

Most notably, I ran my first trail races this year, and I don't think I'm ever looking back. I cannot wait to get back out there on the trails!

It is a quick run this morning. Boy, are my toes sore. I've got one black and blue toe and two on each foot are tender. I think that officially makes me a real runner now! And... another run in the books. Happy about that!

SIGN UP FOR A RACE!

There is nothing like a race to put a flag in the ground for some training and goals. Plus they're fun and a great way to feel part of the bigger running community. Or...**volunteer to assist at a race.**

I have lost many an hour down the rabbit hole that is **UltraSignup**, a clearinghouse of trail races that boggles the mind. There are so many amazing distances, locations, and races to choose from. I particularly love learning about beautiful places to run that I've never heard of, even though they're not far from home.

For road races, **RunningintheUSA** is my "go to" source. Of course, after you run a few of these you end up on race director mailing lists. I have a separate email inbox for the all the awesome race announcements I get these days.

DAY 335. TUESDAY, APRIL 5. PORTLAND, OR

As I geek out on UltraSignup and obsess over the possibilities of some of these races, I've been studying the elevation gains.

I remind myself that the brutal staircases in my neighborhood gain less than 100 feet in elevation and that many of these races have thousands and thousands of feet in elevation gain. Yikes. As a sidenote—the elevation gain for the Barkley marathon is 66,000 feet—that's like climbing Mt. Everest... twice! While I don't necessarily aspire to that, I do aspire to longer and more challenging trail runs and want to be prepared for that elevation so I am being mindful of that now and throwing hills into my runs more often.

My quads are still feeling the hill climbing from Sunday's trail race during the first mile this morning but after that I mostly forget about them. Also, pollen is in the air. Lots and lots of pollen. Yellow powdery stuff is covering everything and I notice my voice has dropped an octave when I return from running. I suppose this too shall pass.

DAY 336. WEDNESDAY, APRIL 6. PORTLAND, OR

I read on one of my runner groups yesterday that a simple way to work on getting faster is to run on the track—fast on the straightaways and a regular pace around the curves. I'm not sure I'll ever get so technical about my speed workouts that I'll be timing them, and this feels like an uncomplicated way to make it happen.

This afternoon is Shea's first meet on the track and field team. As I am doing my version of the speed workout on the same track these athletes will be running on later today, I am taking my hat off to them. Pushing yourself all out on the track in front of a bunch of people is no joke. Good luck later today, *everyone*!

DAY 337. THURSDAY, APRIL 7. PORTLAND, OR

This week is highlighting for me how excellent of a stress reliever running can be. It's been a really challenging few weeks, and running helps me keep my head screwed on straight and my energy even. I think about stuff while I'm out there, and I often get some of my best ideas. If only I could remember them all!

DAY 338. FRIDAY, APRIL 8. PORTLAND, OR

Trails, I am coming for you! It's efficient to hit the road right outside my front door, but, boy, I miss the dirt!

COMPRESSION SOCKS

Yes or no? Some people say they really work wonders. Others think those claims are full of it. I donned them this morning and my legs felt great—ready to rock it. It seems like for some time afterwards though that my legs were tingling and pinging, like the blood flow had some recalibrating to do. Many people swear by them, not for running, but afterwards for recovery. I like them, but my jury is still out on the benefits.

DAY 339. SATURDAY, APRIL 9. PORTLAND, OR

This has been a very full, compressed and stressful time yet my blood pressure is so low my doctor said, "Hello, hello?

Anyone in there?" when checking it this week. I chalk this up to my daily miles and believe this would be a very different story were I not committed to my running practice and taking care of myself well.

Another longer weekend run today with lots of thoughts circulating and things getting worked out in my mind. Thank God, I get to run!

TIP: The American Heart Association says regular running can reduce or prevent high blood pressure, and they should know!

DAY 340. SUNDAY, APRIL 10. PORTLAND, OR

Love, love, love Sunday morning runs and their spaciousness. There is not a single car on the streets this morning. It's a beautiful sunrise and a great way to start the day before heading out to the airport.

I'm producing an annual conference—our big public event for the year. Where I'm going, the days are long with epically early mornings, the weather is snowy (it's warm and springlike here) and running outside isn't much of an option—parking lots and busy streets without sidewalks so...it looks like a dreadmill week ahead. When I was at the same hotel last year, I ran on a treadmill and could not believe how warm I got. It was winter, and I was accustomed to my morning runs in 30-degree weather. An indoor run in the gym where it was about 70 degrees didn't actually make me feel that great, but I'm grateful it's there and that I have an easy option. Maybe this time I will turn down the gym thermostat!

This morning I vowed that when I return from my trip I will get in more runs on the trails. Need that!

DAY 341. MONDAY, APRIL 11. CHICAGO, IL

I was working with my leadership program coach the other day on the importance of letting complaints out—perhaps in a rant style—in order to move past them toward solution.

So here's my running rant this morning:

- There are no treadmills available when I get to the gym. Oh great...waiting.
- The first one that comes available is from the sweatiest guy in the place. He asks me to wait while he wipes it down. Oh, that makes it feel a lot cleaner—not! Ew!
- There's a mirror not a foot in front of the treadmill so all there is to look at is my face as it gets more and more red, because...
- It's so hot in here! People come and work out. They get warmer. Why is it so hot in here to begin with?!
- Each time I push the elevation gain button the treadmill shuts down. Start, stop, start, stop.
- The picture on the treadmill screen is of a mountain I'm supposed to be "climbing" during my run. Since the elevation isn't working, the little red dot on the screen that represents me runs back and forth across the bottom of the mountain but never gets to go up it. The visual is like one of those nightmares you have when you run as fast as you can but can't ever get anywhere.

Now that that's out of the way:

- I never run with my headphones on outside because it just makes me feel unsafe. I love music, and I can listen this morning while I'm on the treadmill, so I do.

- I like the camaraderie of the other folks in the gym—even if we don't exchange any words.
- I have a huge day in front of me, and this run will help my baseline stay calm, cool, and collected.
- No matter what, any day I run, no matter where, is better than any day I don't.
- I'm grateful I get to run today!

DAY 342. TUESDAY, APRIL 12. CHICAGO, IL

I show up at the gym early this morning dressed for the steamy indoor temperature. I have an early morning meeting and need to be efficient. I got up at 2:00 a.m. Portland time to make it work. And…the hotel is big, the gym is small, and it is packed with not a treadmill available in sight. What to do…it's 30 degrees and I head outside in a thin t-shirt and shorts. And, that's how I end up running really fast through a neighborhood of one-story brick houses near the freeway and the airport. A girl's got to do what a girl's got to do.

Today is our opening day, and I emceed the conference. It was a huge day with lots of stage time for me and lots of details and I really needed to be on. I felt fueled and grounded and confident and happy, and I attribute so much of that presence to my running practice. Amen.

DAY 343. WEDNESDAY, APRIL 13. CHICAGO, IL

There's a nature preserve across a busy road from my hotel. I run over to it this morning, but it is just getting light out and the forest is dark. I don't need to remind myself too hard that while this is nature—it is nature in the middle of a city, a big city not known for its lack of crime, a city I don't know well. As much as I am so ready to get on a trail in some trees, it really isn't a safe or a sound idea. I find an open field and run around and around it. At one point I step into a hole up to my shin and remarkably and thankfully don't twist anything. I cross back over the busy street and run around some parking lots and streets filled with big trucks. Crazy and disjointed as it is, it gets the blood pumping and the fresh air into the lungs, though I am already ready to get back home to the streets and trails of Portland!

DAY 344. THURSDAY, APRIL 14. CHICAGO, IL

From my upper story hotel window I spot what looks like a well-lit road that runs alongside part of the perimeter of the nature preserve. A run alongside some trees is better than a run alongside no trees, so I cross four lanes, then four lanes again to get there only to discover the "road" is only a parking lot—a semi-creepy one at that. I run back across those eight lanes and into a parking lot where I commence to run around and around and around on the blacktop.

As I was in the airport later in the evening I saw a woman whose body I can only describe as curiously misshapen walking laboriously towards the elevator as the crowds rushed to the escalator. Witnessing her reminded me of how incredibly grateful I am to be able to run, to walk, to move my body— whether that is in an airport, a parking lot, on the road or trail, or just anywhere.

A healthy body is a sacred thing and I honor that—even if I sound like an ass when I say that, I mean it!

DAY 345. FRIDAY, APRIL 15. PORTLAND, OR

It's so good to be home! My time zone and eating habits and just about everything are off from these last five days away, and I am so happy to get out in the fresh air, to see friendly faces and to have endless choices for routes—all of which have some trees, grass, bushes, flowers, even when I'm running in the street. I love Portland, love my family, love my dogs, and love running here with all of that!

DAY 346. SATURDAY, APRIL 16. PORTLAND, OR

Lingo alert! Ever heard of negative splits? That's when the time it takes to complete each mile during your run is faster than the one before it. Many times runners, particularly in a race, go out fast at a pace that can't be maintained throughout their run. Negative splits, however, illustrate that you've still got gas in the tank at the end of the run. That is what happened during my run today, and it is an awesome feeling!

During the run today I thought a lot about my time in Chicago this week. It is an enormous job to be both the producer and the emcee of an event—so many balls in the air, so many things to think about, so many people to connect with, so much going on behind the scenes, and the need to show up on stage with the presence to say the right things in the right way at the right time.

Over the course of our days together numerous—and I mean really a lot—of people came up to me to tell me how much they appreciate my presence on stage. That it makes them feel calm, Zen, peaceful, at ease, in control....I have always carried a calm presence in the face of a lot going on, but I really think that all of this is supported by the fact that my blood pressure is very low thanks to genetics, good self-care, and…running.

Running helps me do the other things in my life better. Mic drop.

DAY 347. SUNDAY, APRIL 17. PORTLAND, OR

Jeff has been on my mind so much lately. Yesterday I was thinking about stage presence and how Jeff just had it in spades. He had this stance that he would take on stage—a sort of peaceful and grounded but "try to take me down and I'll flatten you" kind of stance. He had so many practices that fueled his presence. He used to run a bit, and we hiked together on numerous occasions. His birthday is coming up soon and I just think about him a lot on my runs and all of the time, really. Once I'm a mile or so into my runs and I get settled and after I've gone through the to do list for the day in my head, everything in my mind opens up and that's where it goes. So grateful for that space.

The weather is really warm now and there are more people out at 8:00 a.m. than I have seen in a long time. It's the change of the seasons…again.

DAY 348. MONDAY, APRIL 18. PORTLAND, OR

If you are losing faith in human nature,
go out and watch a marathon.
—Katharine Switzer,
First woman to run the Boston Marathon
as a numbered entry

By the time I am out of bed this morning the Boston Marathon has already begun. I just love watching these races on the screen, and the whole time I am out for my morning miles I'm inspired knowing they're out there at the same time giving it their all. I particularly loved the story of one runner whose father wasn't in the room the day she was born because he was out running the Boston Marathon, and here she is 26 years later on that same course—and aiming for the 2020 Olympic marathon team, too.

And how about Bobbi Gibb, the first woman to ever complete the marathon?! If you can believe it, when she ran for the first time in 1966, women were not allowed to register officially so she had to sneak into the race. Today, she is the grand marshal. That was only 50 years ago! My, how things have changed and how far we still have to go! So grateful for all the runners who have come before to make this sport what it is today!

DAY 349. TUESDAY, APRIL 19. PORTLAND, OR

Shea was home sick from school yesterday, and the thing most on our minds was getting better so he could run at his meet this week—and dialing in the different scenarios of how well you have to be in order to run and perform. Speaking of, since he wasn't eating much yesterday somehow neither did I and…I'm really feeling it during my run this morning. I love how a giant bowl of spaghetti at night makes me feel ready to roll in the morning. Yesterday's smoothies and soup just didn't really cut the mustard. Still, it is a beautiful morning for a slower-than-usual run leading into another hot day. So grateful I get to run today!

Also, I pulled up all of the paperwork I'll need to send in to make my membership in the US Running Streak Association official come day 366—17 days, baby!

DAY 350. WEDNESDAY, APRIL 20. PORTLAND, OR

Wow. 350 days. Listen and you can hear the sound of me patting myself on the back. Really, only 16 days until I've reached the year mark?! So much to reflect on.

One thing that's really got my attention now is time. I was able to make daily running a habit because banging out a mile didn't take much time. The longer the distance the longer the amount of time you need to commit to for getting your miles in. When I first started my streak I had days where I ran for 10 minutes. These days I am averaging half an hour or more a day. I notice two things about that: if I had started out this streak committing to 30 minutes of running a day all manner of excuses would have befallen me. The commitment would have been too much. The other thing I know is that I wish it could be more time! There are mornings I wish I could run for an hour or more, and I have to juggle the impact on my sleep, family time or work meetings. Add to it that the more I run on the roads the more I crave the trails—which, unfortunately, are not right outside my front door like the road is. So, I have to get myself there.

Still, half an hour doesn't feel like that much. It's really not. But at the end of the week, that usually adds up to about five hours of running a week. In some ways that still doesn't sound like much at all but on the other hand…

PROGRESS REPORT: If someone had asked me at the beginning of this challenge if I had four to five hours a week to commit to a project I would have definitely said, "No way." Yet here I am running at least that much each week. Funny how the streak can allow these things to sneak up on you!

I'm also acutely aware there are some people for whom my weekly time is what they might put in in a day. Trail runs can take hours—amazing, wonderful, satisfying, challenging hours. That's not where I'm at right now, but it is a place I am aiming. For now, juggling a full-time job and a full-time family and life, this is what is working for me.

The fact that I have stuck with this every single day
for almost a year tells me something is right about it.

And, it still opens my mind to so many more possibilities of what else I might accomplish if I were to approach it like this—just a little bit every day instead of my typical all-in dive in and then burn out.

THE ONLINE RUNNING COMMUNITY ROCKS!

You can find **Streak Runners International** and the **United States Streak Running Association** online. On their websites you can view the current rosters of streak runners and have your mind blown by the length of some of the streaks. Simply heroic!

In addition, the Facebook page for Streak Runners International is lit up day and night by people logging in with news from their runs and races, advice seekers, advice givers, company for mourning when a streak comes to an end and folks cheering for those who get out there every day, no matter the odds. There are people who run just the minimum mile and those who go long, long, long distances. They're all there.

Similarly, the Facebook group for the **Trail and Ultra-Running** community is a hotbed of activity, awesomeness, badassery, and snark. Join at your own risk.

DAY 351. THURSDAY, APRIL 21. PORTLAND, OR

I'm still lazy. Now that the weather is getting warmer there are all kinds of people doing all manner of workouts in the park in the morning. I run past the folks on the pull-up bars, the bootcamp that meets on the field, and the coaches running their team through extra training this morning. Me? I just put one foot in front of the other. Some days it's faster than others. Some days there are hills or stairs or intervals. But mostly, I just go. It's not heroic or terribly exciting or even that hard. For now, it is enough for me.

However…I'm obsessing over the races on UltraSignup! I want to do so many of them. There are tons of choices if you want to run 50K, 50 miles or more, even a 200 miler, races on Mt. St. Helens (I've climbed it and it is amazing, but racing—wow!) and an awesome three-day circumnavigation of Mt. Rainier race. Clearly I'm not there yet—did you see that previous thing about still being lazy?! You can't be lazy if you're going to prepare for one of these things.

And…one of the ways to prepare is to get some elevation in. We have a few hills around my neighborhood but they are sure as heck not the same as running up a mountain. That kind of training requires a whole new level of commitment. Like yesterday one 25k I got kind of excited about recommends that you come and run the course in advance because it's so humbling. That means doing it twice and then some. Hmmm…I aspire but yet hesitate in putting a plan in action. I'm so damned happy to remain injury free and to just get out there every day. On the other hand, I know magic waits on the other side once I commit. Sigh.

DAY 352. FRIDAY, APRIL 22. PORTLAND, OR

I have to admit I walked in the door this morning feeling like somewhat of a badass for being thoroughly drenched from head to toe. It rained all night and the trees and flowers have just gone berzerkers in my neighborhood. It's so lush and green, and it didn't really start pouring until the last mile. A nice warm spring rain to make the flowers grow. I'll take it!

This is how I know the running streak does a number on my psyche, because a week of beautiful weather interrupted by a dark day of heavy rain would usually bum me out. Instead, I'm practically skipping around, nicely infused with endorphins and viewing the day through a different, happier lens. Lower blood pressure too. And only a little smug.

DAY 353. SATURDAY, APRIL 23. PORTLAND, OR

I took some advice I saw on the Trail and Ultra-Running Facebook group page and decided to pay no attention to my pace or distance today, I'm just running for a set amount of time—an hour. After a bit I look at my watch and see that I'm 43 minutes in and the thought of 17 more minutes is no big deal. In fact, at 60 I feel like I could just kept going—and so I do.

PROGRESS REPORT: An hour of running without stopping was no big deal. Not all that long ago, it would have been.

It's amazing what happens even just one mile away from home, too, as I'm running down streets I've never been on before seeing beautiful homes and gardens. Just one mile from home puts me in some unknown territory.

TIP: Running is such an enjoyable way to explore new places— even in your own backyard!

DAY 354. SUNDAY, APRIL 24. PORTLAND, OR

Love my Sunday rundays—nice and easy and long with lots of time for reflection and taking in the beautiful spring scenery.

Running really is my meditation. For years I beat myself up for not being able to keep up with a regular sitting meditation practice. Meditation is something that, when I did manage to get my practice in, I invariably felt better afterwards. Yet although I'd participated in plenty of retreats and even lived for a time across the street from a well-known meditation center, for all the times I launched into a regular practice, my zafus (pillows for sitting meditation) sit mostly untouched.

The thing that has changed is that I used to really beat myself up about it. I'm not hard on myself about this any longer because I get my meditation in everyday—it's just out on the road or the trail or even on the treadmill instead of on the pillow. I focus on my breath. My mind wanders. I solve problems and come up with new creative ideas. I come back to my breath.

I think a lot about Jeff and about Kevin and my Dad. I talk to them all. I know that each one of them would have gotten a kick out of this practice. Somehow, when I am running I feel like I can be present with each one of them, instead of being present to their loss.

Running can be a time to reflect and grieve and show gratitude—all of those things. It is a moving meditation.

DAY 355. MONDAY, APRIL 25. PORTLAND, OR

Putting a flag in the ground by signing up for a race is an audacious thing to do. I've run more than 20 5k road races with my family over the last few years now. These have mostly been of the big community variety with thousands of runners. We have plenty of those to choose from here in Portland, and we do a handful each year.

More and more I am less attracted to those (though several will always hold a place in my heart) and really just want to get out there on the trails. I have a whole slew of races coming up now—the summer series in Forest Park (five evening races five weeks in a row on different courses in Forest Park, the largest urban forest in the United States), a small handful of 5ks in the park (no pavement, all trail), and a couple of others in beautiful locations as I aspire to greater and greater distances in places I've never explored before. As they say, the longer run puts the tiger in the cat! Oregon is amazing for this. I may not live on a trail system, but nearby there are forests and waterfalls and deserts that are all calling my name! And, perusing the races on UltraSignup is like being sucked down the rabbithole! Geez…the options!

The theme of this morning's run is "noticing." Noticing little pings in my knee and in my feet that are most likely a little payback for an increase in pavement miles over the weekend. It's nothing to be alarmed about right now; it's just important to notice and to take corrective action if need be. Being out on the road or trail or track gives you lots of opportunity to notice!

TIP: When I was marathon training I would keep Dixie cups full of frozen water to take out and rub along my shins after long runs to help keep the shin splints at bay.

DAY 356. TUESDAY, APRIL 26. PORTLAND, OR

Today is my old friend, colleague, collaborator, partner Jeff's birthday. Like today, I don't think a single other run has gone by this year when I haven't thought of him. Happy birthday, pal. I miss you.

DAY 357. WEDNESDAY, APRIL 27. PORTLAND, OR

It's my third day in a row of running to and then around and around the track to run on a more forgiving surface. I think my shins are thanking me. On the downside there are no hills, but on the upside it provides an easier opportunity to work on speed. Even though we just go around…and around—like the outdoor version of the treadmill, I like the camaraderie at the track, and this time of year there are more and more people coming out.

There's one guy I see often on the track or on the road. He's very tall with legs that end at my shoulders and just a gorgeous runner. I imagine he is probably a professional athlete. When I ran with Calliope at the track one time he was there. She sprinted around one of the inner lanes while he ran around the outer. She was proud of herself to have won a "race" against him—one that he didn't even know he was running. Now, every time I see him, I think of him as her racing nemesis in a comedic kind of way—this guy two or three times her age and height. Maybe you had to be there, but it makes me laugh—and in some strange way helps her aspire too.

PROGRESS REPORT: Just a week until I've completed a year of running! I am doing a good job of impressing myself.

DAY 358. THURSDAY, APRIL 28. PORTLAND, OR

I'm running another trail race this weekend and want to get in some elevation action to help prepare, so I'm going for a stair run…up the staircase, an eighth of a mile to the next staircase, down the staircase, an eighth of a mile to the next, up the staircase, eighth of a mile, etc., etc. in a continual loop for about an hour.

Today I'm really tuned in to my breath. I love that rhythmic breathing. I often sing songs in my head while I run along to that rhythm. The other creatures that make a rhythmic sound this time of day are the chickens waking up around the neighborhood. It is true what they say about Portland's urban farmers. I pass about a dozen backyard coops on my loops today. Bock. Bock. Bock.

One thing I think about while huffing up and down is my gym membership. Yes, I have one. Have I been once in the last year? I don't think so. I hang on to it because when I have used it consistently for yoga classes it costs me as much for a month as it would for about a class and a half at the yoga studio and, somehow, letting it go closes the door on the possibility of getting back into yoga. I do aspire to get back to yoga. Maybe it's time to take another 30-day challenge!

DAY 359. FRIDAY, APRIL 29. PORTLAND, OR

As I approach one year of my running streak I am struck that in some ways this has not been *that* hard to accomplish. Many days the most difficult part has just been lacing up and getting out the door. Thanks to the slow build, running has really become part of my routine—it's just one of the many things that I do every day like brushing my teeth. It has become routine for me, and it has become routine for the people around me.

In fact, the people around me, namely my family, are kicking butt with their own running. Matt has joined me on as many days as he could this year, and has done plenty on his own, as well. He struggles with injury prevention, likely a holdover from many years of playing competitive tennis, but is getting stronger all the time. Shea kicked butt during his first high school cross country season and is loving his time on the track and field team right now. He is so determined. Calliope, who has never fully embraced distance running, is coming into her own as a shorter distance competitor in her first season on the middle school track and field team now, too, and is slaying the competition in the 400 meter race.

Already two nights this week we spent time replaying video of both kids at their meets, examining their form and celebrating the experience on the big screen. I'm so proud of everyone!

TIP: Perhaps nothing quite evidences our family's involvement in the sport better than the Sisyphean mountain of laundry that we accumulate on a daily basis. Talk about a workout! Don't let it pile up too long lest that stank sets in and never goes away!

This morning's run was routine...and enjoyable. The enjoyable days still way outweigh the struggle days.

I have never once regretted getting out for my daily run. Not once. BOOM!

DAY 360. SATURDAY, APRIL 30.
WILLAMETTE MISSION TRAIL CHALLENGE. SALEM, OR

Ughaiyeeeearghphack! That sound has interrupted my trail run reverie repeatedly this morning. Simply put, that is the sound of someone sliding into a patch of mud, arms windmilling forwards, then backwards, as their equilibrium rotates around until they are either flat on their ass or find themselves hurtling forward again towards another patch.

Today was my second trail race, and here are a few things I learned:

- When the race organizers say there's a bit of mud out there, "bit" is a relative term.

- Also, that bit of mud *will* splash up into your open mouth.
- Tie your shoes just a little bit tighter when going out on said runs with a bit of mud lest you risk losing them to the bog.
- Remember that you are out there to enjoy the scenery but take your eyes off the trail at your own risk.
- It feels as good to hear "good job" from a fellow runner as it does to say it to another one.
- Running a race with a friend makes it that much more enjoyable.
- A post-race beer is like a gift from the angels.

That was so much fun. When can I do it again?!

DAY 361. SUNDAY, MAY 1. PORTLAND, OR

I'm still feeling the high from yesterday's trail run on the most beautiful morning today—it's just starting to get warm and breezy. It's our wedding anniversary and after so many years the thing we still love to do together most is any kind of outdoor adventure. We run to meet up with family and friends at the park and then walk our way to breakfast afterwards. So happy to be alive this morning and to have this healthy way to celebrate it all.

DAY 362. MONDAY, MAY 2. PORTLAND, OR

I'm a terrible afternoon runner. I get side stiches. I feel like a slug. I get too warm and uncomfortable. And…apparently, I complain too.

Sometimes life calls for changing the routine so…today's run ended up a slow, hot run through the neighborhood, viewing the tiny daisies sprouting in the grass.

DAY 363. TUESDAY, MAY 3. PORTLAND, OR

TIP: That extra five or 10 minutes you spend under the covers while the alarm is going off would be way better spent out on your run. You're welcome.

DAY 364. WEDNESDAY, MAY 4. PORTLAND, OR

This morning's run is just lovely. I'm not checking my pace, time or distance and instead am just running through the neighborhood in the early morning. It rained last night and everything seems to have grown. It is quiet and still and so beautiful with everything in bloom. I work out a few things in my head and give attention to some other things. I think about people I miss and give thanks for the things I often take for granted.

Running helps me quiet my mind and tunes me in to my little role in this big thing called life. Yep.

DAY 365. THURSDAY, MAY 5. PORTLAND, OR

Little by little a little becomes a lot.
—Tanzanian proverb

It feels like my birthday when I wake up today. I jump out of bed at dark o'clock and head out. Okay, maybe I don't actually jump, but I'm moving with some extra *umph* like I'm the holder of a special secret. Outside, the morning is mild and peaceful and on this run, like so many, I am reflective.

When I set out 365 days ago to attempt to run a mile a day every day for 30 days, truly I had no idea it would lead to this moment. I'd never heard of this kind of streaking and had no idea there was this amazing community of streak runners, all over the world, who have dedicated themselves to their health, fitness, growth, development, and their incredible support for one another.

I also had no idea I was capable of such a deep commitment to something that, while it serves me and the others around me so well, in many ways is all about me. I couldn't have known what it might be like to stick to this commitment no matter what was going on, where I might find myself or how I might be feeling. I just didn't know what I didn't know. I had to create it.

I wondered for weeks whether this day's run, the one that makes one year of my running complete, would be dramatic and exiting or anticlimactic. It's not really either. I ran a handful of miles through my neighborhood, around the park and back like I'd done so many other times this year. No speedwork, no hills, no company…just an easy run. Today's run isn't anything extraordinary which, I have learned, seems to be the way when you commit to something with such relentless consistency. This run, however, as part of that unwavering commitment to my running streak is a crucial brick in the wall of building something extraordinary—a solid, consistent, satisfying, growth-builder of an experiment I am committed to Every.Single.Day.

For all the other streakers, my family who has supported me to get here, for all my unfolding and discoveries and for every literal step of the way here, I am so terrifically grateful.

Along the path in the park I find some chalk writing. It has an arrow pointing to the path and says, "You go, girl!" I believe I will. Streak on!

CHAPTER FOUR

THE FINISH LINE

Out on the roads, there is fitness and self-discovery
and the persons we were destined to be.
—George Sheehan, running legend

I was milling about before a trail race recently when the race
director called out: "Runners to the starting line!" As I made
my way over, I couldn't help thinking that it wasn't exactly
the starting line. I mean, there was so much that had come
before this moment—all the early mornings, the miles, the
time, nutrition, gear, and the literal blood, sweat, and tears,
especially the sweat! I thought perhaps, at least in my mind,
a more apt thing to do was to call it the continuation line.

I feel similar about the finish line. It may be the end of
that particular race, but it's not the end at all, just a new place
to start from.

Similarly, the end of the year in which I have run Every. Single.Day. for 365 days feels like just the beginning. There are so many people in front of me who have passed 365 days and kept on going. I want to be in their club. Even as I run primarily solo, I appreciate all the runners who have come before and all the runners who run now…and all those miles! Similarly, I appreciate all of those who can't run, people who don't and maybe never will. They are one of the reasons so many of us say, "Thank God I got to run today!"

I surprised myself with how relatively easy this challenge has been for me. I had a decent base to start from, but in some ways, it really wasn't about the running at all.

Running was the Trojan horse of goodness that ushered in a shift for me, the shift I was hoping to find when I committed to a year of 30-day challenges. I was looking to get my mojo back. I found it. I still lose it sometimes, but it's mostly back. I found some other things too. I found consistency and discipline. I remembered how to build a foundation. I set a goal and I blew it out of the water. It has allowed me to keep asking myself how many other places there are in my life where I might be able to do that too. That's not something I was thinking about 365 days ago.

All year long I have managed to remain injury free. I credit a sane and reasonable approach to my distance, time, and pace. When I started, I was doing the minimum of about seven miles a week. I took a whole year to move to a place of about 30 miles per week now. There are plenty of runners I've experienced this last year for whom my weekly mileage is their daily. I may get there someday, too, but I'm perfectly happy where I am at this moment. My blood pressure is low, my weight is stable, I feel fit and stronger, and I can really relish tucking into a mountain of food and beer!

Over the course of this year, like so many others, I have covered a lot of ground. I've run in a number of different states and a few countries. I've run in the warm sand, in the deep snow, and in rain that came down sideways in icy sheets. I've run in hotel gyms across the country, inside an airport, on a boat, on an empty stomach, and after a huge meal. I've run while on vacation, on my birthday, on Thanksgiving and Christmas and Hanukkah, and every single holiday that comes in a year. I've run while drunk, while feeling strong, and while feeling really sick and awful. I've run with my husband and with my kids, with thousands of others in races, and mostly, by myself. I've spent a lot of miles reflecting, thinking, meditating, smiling, and crying.

Running every single damned day has taught me consistency and sticktoitiveness. I understand what dedication to a personal practice *really* means now, and I know what it takes to do something no matter what. And now that I've done that it somehow has become less of a big deal and more of something that I just do. Sometimes it's the best hour of the day. Most often it's harder to get out the door than it is to do the actual running.

I've been inspired by so many people this year in the running community, both those who run unimaginably long distances and those who are just huffing their way around the block. I have a particularly soft spot in my heart for the runners who have overcome incredible adversity just to get their butts out there, and for those who have lost volumes of weight in the process or moved away from drugs or alcohol—wow. More power to you!

Runners are hands down the most supportive, encouraging, friendly, and crazy bunch out there. They cheer each other on, celebrate successes, and are there for each other when injury strikes or a streak comes to an end. They know that every day can be a good day when you run. And boy, do they run!

I love that as I have continued to run, the itch to run more gets itchier. There are so many places to go—both literally and figuratively—and so many experiences to look forward to, even if that just means getting out the door day after day.

As my old pal Jeff used to say, "Just keep moving." And, that is what I intend to do.

ACKNOWLEDGMENTS

Tim Ferriss for providing the inspiration to begin my year of my "middle-aged mom with a full-time job in a slump try this at home" 30-day challenges. Also, I'm glad you have a dog now!

Dr. Ray McClanahan is the man! He and his staff at Northwest Foot and Ankle, home of Correct Toes, have kept me running. Thank you, thank you for your pioneering philosophy and for taking such good care of so many feats...er, feets.

Tim Levy who wrote the *Fast Book Handbook*, which convinced me that getting a book out the door didn't have to be such a big, fat, hairy deal after all. And, thanks for the introduction to Tim, Eli Call.

Big thanks to Todd Kushner, Robyn Tenenbaum, and my sisters, Jeanne Rodgers and Liz van Amerongen, who all read early versions of this book and assured me that while perhaps it wasn't as lame as my sixth grade diary, it wasn't as mortifying either. Those stories are for another book.

Matt played a starring role both in and out of the story. Without his support there are many days I wouldn't have gotten out the door for a run. In addition to joining me side by side for so many runs, he has taken a bullet for the team more often than I can count by taking on the family morning routine while I was out on a run or holding my luggage so I could run in an airport or chauffeuring us to a race. He is my biggest cheerleader and the wind beneath my running shoes, even after I shooed him off the trail during my first trail race!

I'm so happy to have shared so many runs with my kids, Shea and Calliope. They have both developed into beautiful track and cross country athletes of their own, and I could not be more proud, much as it embarrasses them for me to tell you so.

Mark Washburne who runs the United States Running Association and Streak Runners International certifying runners for membership once they have passed the first-year mark of their streak. Thanks for being the glue for this inspiring community!

All of the runners in the Streak Running International community who share their stories and cheer each other on every running step of the way. You guys are my heroes!

In my newfound love of running I think I may have also found a home in the Trail and Ultra Running community (TAUR), if they'll have me.

For all the others who help keep this amazing running community humming—the race organizers, volunteers, local running stores, and all the other people who support us—and most of all for those who lace up and get out there and RUN. Godspeed to you all.